MEDICAL INTELLIGENCE UNIT

EXERCISE IMMUNOLOGY

Bente Klarlund Pedersen, M.D., Ph.D.
The Copenhagen Muscle Research Center
and Department of Infectious Diseases
University of Copenhagen
Copenhagen, Denmark

Springer
New York Berlin Heidelberg London Paris
Tokyo Hong Kong Barcelona Budapest

R.G. LANDES COMPANY
AUSTIN

MEDICAL INTELLIGENCE UNIT
EXERCISE IMMUNOLOGY

R.G. LANDES COMPANY
Austin, Texas, U.S.A.

Printed in the U.S.A.

Please address all inquiries to the Publishers:
R.G. Landes Company, 810 S. Church Street, Georgetown, Texas, U.S.A. 78626
Phone: 512/ 863 7762; FAX: 512/ 863 0081

International distributor (except North America):
Springer-Verlag GmbH & Co. KG
Tiergartenstrasse 17, D-69121 Heidelberg, Germany

Springer

International ISBN: 3-540-62039-7

While the authors, editors and publisher believe that drug selection and dosage and the specifications and usage of equipment and devices, as set forth in this book, are in accord with current recommendations and practice at the time of publication, they make no warranty, expressed or implied, with respect to material described in this book. In view of the ongoing research, equipment development, changes in governmental regulations and the rapid accumulation of information relating to the biomedical sciences, the reader is urged to carefully review and evaluate the information provided herein.

Library of Congress Cataloging-in-Publication Data

Pedersen, Bente Klarlund, 1956—
Exercise immunology / Bente Klarlund Pedersen
p. cm. — (Medical intelligence unit)
Includes bibliographical references and index.
ISBN 0-57059-420-1 (alk. paper)
1. Exercise—Immunological aspects. I. Title . II. Series.
[DNLM: 1. Exercise—physiology. 2. Immunity QT 255 P371e 1997]
616.5'21—dc20
DNLM/DLC
for Library of Congress

96-45260
CIP

Publisher's Note

R.G. Landes Company publishes six book series: *Medical Intelligence Unit, Molecular Biology Intelligence Unit, Neuroscience Intelligence Unit, Tissue Engineering Intelligence Unit, Biotechnology Intelligence Unit* and *Environmental Intelligence Unit.* The authors of our books are acknowledged leaders in their fields and the topics are unique. Almost without exception, no other similar books exist on these topics.

Our goal is to publish books in important and rapidly changing areas of bioscience and environment for sophisticated researchers and clinicians. To achieve this goal, we have accelerated our publishing program to conform to the fast pace in which information grows in bioscience. Most of our books are published within 90 to 120 days of receipt of the manuscript. We would like to thank our readers for their continuing interest and welcome any comments or suggestions they may have for future books.

Shyamali Ghosh
Publications Director
R.G. Landes Company

Dedication

To my parents

CONTENTS

EDITOR

Bente Klarlund Pedersen, M.D., Ph.D.
The Copenhagen Muscle Research Center
and Department of Infectious Diseases
RHIMA Center, Rigshospitalet
University of Copenhagen
Copenhagen, Denmark

CONTRIBUTORS

Helle Bruunsgaard, M.D.
The Copenhagen Muscle Research Center and Department of Infectious Diseases
RHIMA Center, Rigshospitalet
University of Copenhagen
Copenhagen, Denmark
Chapters 6,10

Inge Haunstrup Clemmensen, M.D.
Danish Cancer Society
Division for Cancer Epidemiology
Copenhagen, Denmark
Chapter 11

Mogens Kappel, M.D.
The Copenhagen Muscle Research Center and Department of Infectious Diseases
RHIMA Center, Rigshospitalet
University of Copenhagen
Copenhagen, Denmark
Chapter 3, 4

Mads Klokker, M.D.
The Copenhagen Muscle Research Center and Department of Infectious Diseases
RHIMA Center, Rigshospitalet
University of Copenhagen
Copenhagen, Denmark
Chapters 3, 4

Henning Bay Nielsen, M.D.
The Copenhagen Muscle Research Center and Department of Infectious Diseases
RHIMA Center, Rigshospitalet
University of Copenhagen
Copenhagen, Denmark
Chapter 2

CONTRIBUTORS

Thomas Rohde, M.D.
The Copenhagen Muscle Research Center and Department of Infectious Diseases
RHIMA Center, Rigshospitalet
University of Copenhagen
Copenhagen, Denmark
Chapter 5, 6

Henrik Ullum, M.D.
The Copenhagen Muscle Research Center and Department of Infectious Diseases
RHIMA Center, Rigshospitalet
University of Copenhagen
Copenhagen, Denmark
Chapter 8

Acknowledgments

My interest in exercise immunology started with the questions of why so much research is available regarding pathophysiology and immunology, or pharmacology and immunology; and why so little knowledge exists about the relationship between normal physiology and immunology? When I began to consider exercise as a prototype of physical stress, I also realized that exercise could be used as a model to study the relationships between the nervous, the endocrine and the immune systems. Furthermore, exercise serves as a useful model in the study of the acute phase response to local injury.

I have used this monograph to step back and look at the progress over the past 10 years. Much has been achieved, although the research in the area of exercise immunology contains many conflicting results. In this book I have tried to generate new models and hypotheses for the underlying mechanisms.

The aim of this book has been to tell a good story. It is also a personal story. I, therefore, invited some of my colleagues in exercise immunology, mostly present or former PhD students in our laboratory, to serve as co-authors. I have tried to cover the various topics in depth. I apologize to those of my colleagues who may not have been adequately mentioned and I can assure them that no malice or arrogance has played a role.

This book could not have been finished had it not been for a number of special people: my co-authors who prepared excellent contributions; Professors Gunnar Bendixen and Vagn Andersen, the Department of Rheumatology, Rigshospitalet, who stimulated my interest in immunology; Professor Peter Skinhøj, The Department of Infectious Diseases, Professor Gunhild Vejlsgaard, The RHIMA center, and Professor Bengt Saltin, The Copenhagen Muscle Research Center, Rigshospitalet, who provided excellent laboratory facilities and stimulated discussions; Professor Ib Lorenzen, the Department of Rheumatology, Hvidovre Hospital, who provided good working conditions and support; Linda Powell, who "polished" my English language; Niels Jørgen Thomsen who gave secretarial assistance; my husband Kim Klarlund who critically read the manuscript and our four children who allowed me to spend more time away from them than usual in order to complete this book. I thank them all wholeheartedly. I also thank the Danish National Research Foundation for support.

CHAPTER 1

Introduction

Bente Klarlund Pedersen

The positive effects of regular exercise are obviously results of a complex interaction between physiological and psychological effects. Thus, it has been shown that exercise can lower blood pressure, improve the lipid profile, enhance mood and decrease sensitivity to pain.[1]

The increasing popularity of regular exercise is probably due to increased public awareness regarding the beneficial effects of exercise on physical and emotional well-being. Many individuals claim that regular exercise increases resistance to infections such as the common cold.[2,3] On the other hand, there have also been anecdotal reports from athletes and their coaches that hard training is associated with increased respiratory tract infections.[2] Today epidemiological evidence exists that supports the anecdotal impression and it has become clear that the function of the immune system is enhanced by moderate physical activity and may be somewhat responsible for exercise-related reduction in illness. In contrast, it has been repeatedly shown that intense exercise causes inhibition of the function of the immune system in the recovery phase following intense exercise.[5]

The first written report on exercise immunology is by Chagrin and Roger[6] who in 1890 reported increased risk of infections in fatigued rats. The first publication in humans on exercise-induced leukocytosis was written by Schultz in 1893.[7] The first publication in English that described "violent leukocytosis" experienced by a small group of runners after the Boston Marathon was reported by Larrabee in 1902.[8]

In the following years, there were only sporadic reports on exercise and immunology, but during the last decade there has been a growing interest in understanding to which degree and by which mechanisms exercise influences the immune system. As a consequence, The International Society of Exercise and Immunology was established in 1993 in Paderborn, Germany, one century after Schulz published his work on exercise-induced leukocytosis.

Today, much research in exercise immunology is stimulated by the acceptance of exercise as a tool to study the immune system. Exercise can be employed as a model for temporary immunosuppression which occurs after severe physical stress. The exercise-stress model can be easily manipulated experimentally, and allows for the study of interactions between the nervous, the endocrine and the immune systems. Furthermore, eccentric exercise which is associated with muscle damage represents a model of the acute phase response to local injury.

This book provides critical reviews of various areas of exercise immunology. Chapter 2 reviews the effects of acute exercise on the immune system in humans. Current views on possible underlying mechanisms are included in chapters 3 through 5. Thus, these chapters discuss the possible roles of neuroendocrine factors; physiological factors, such as hyperthermia and hypoxia, and the possible role of glutamine in exercise-associated immunosuppression. The role of cytokines in the acute phase response to exercise and in exercise-induced muscle damage is discussed in chapter 6. Chapter 7 presents the effect of chronic exercise on resting levels of the immune system. Chapters 8 through 11 deal specifically with the health implications of exercise-induced changes in immune function for infectious diseases, aging, nutrition and cancer.

References

1. Thoren P, Floras JS, Hoffmann P et al. Endorphins and exercise: physiological mechanisms and clinical implications. Med Sci Sports Exerc 1990; 22(4):417-428.
2. Fitzgerald L. Exercise and the immune system. Immunol Today 1988; 9(11):337-339.
3. Nash HL. Can exercise make us immune to disease? Phys Sportsmed 1987; 1:250-253.

4. Nieman DC, Henson DA. Role of endurance exercise in immune senescence. Med Sci Sports Exerc 1994; 26(2):172-181.
5. Hoffman-Goetz L, Pedersen BK. Exercise and the immune system: a model of the stress response? Immunol Today 1994; 15(8):382-7.
6. Charrin, Roger. A L'etude Experimentale du Surmenage; son Influence sur L'infection. Arch de Physiol Norm et Path 1890; 2:273-283.
7. Schultz G. Experimentielle Untersuchungen über das Vorkommen und die diagnostische Bedeutung der Leucocytose. Dtsch Arch Klin Med 1893; 51:234-281.
8. Larrabee RC. Leucocytosis after violent exercise. The J Med Res 1902; 7:76-82.

CHAPTER 2

ACUTE EXERCISE AND THE IMMUNE SYSTEM

Bente Klarlund Pedersen and Henning Bay Nielsen

There are several consistent patterns that emerge regarding leukocyte subpopulations in the blood. The neutrophil concentration increases during exercise and continues to increase postexercise.[1] The lymphocyte concentration increases during exercise and falls below prevalues following intense long-duration exercise (Fig. 2.1).[1] Several reports describe exercise-induced changes in blood mononuclear cells (BMNC).[2-27] The increased lymphocyte concentration is due to the recruitment of all lymphocyte subpopulations to the blood. Thus, both $CD4^+$ T cells, $CD8^+$ T cells, $CD19^+$ B cells, $CD16^+$ natural killer (NK) cells and $CD56^+$ NK cells increase during exercise. Simultaneously, the CD4/CD8 ratio decreases because the CD8 count increases more than the CD4 count. The percentage of $CD4^+$ cells declines primarily due to the fact that the number of NK cells increase more than any other lymphocyte subpopulation. Accordingly, the relative fraction of lymphocyte subpopulations changes (Fig. 2.2).

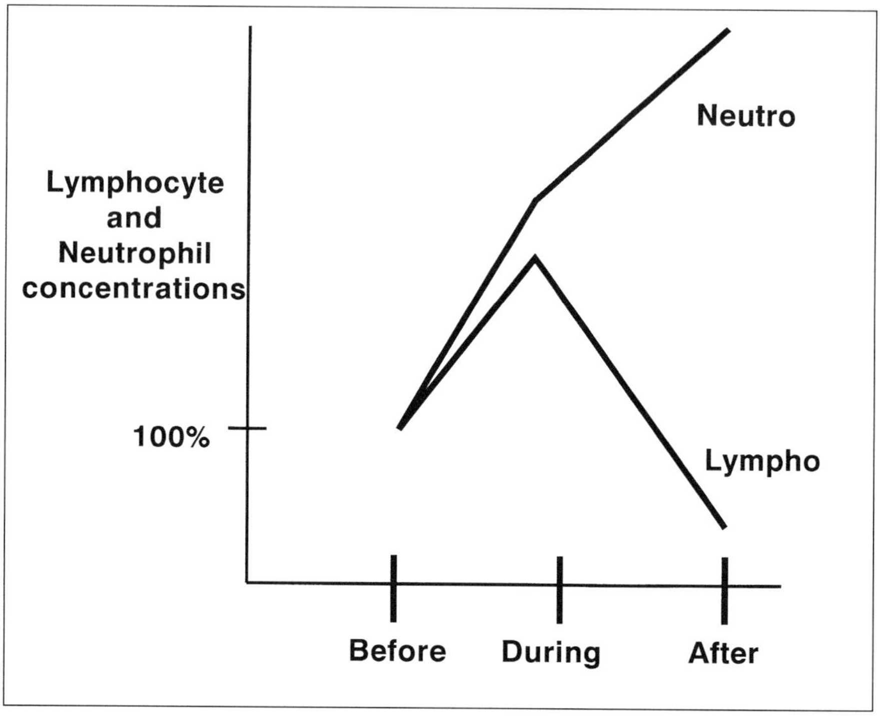

Fig. 2.1. Schematic representation of the changes in concentrations of leukocytes, neutrophils and lymphocytes in relation to acute, intense exercise.

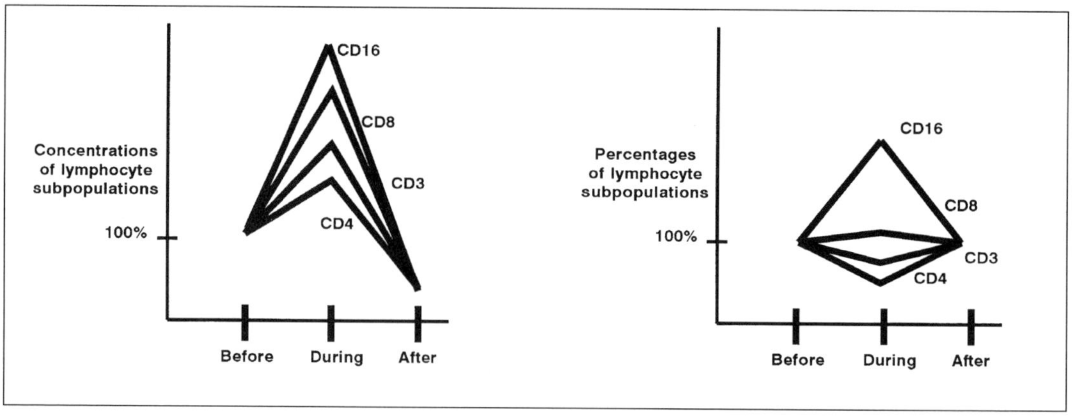

Fig. 2.2. Schematic representation of the changes in concentrations and percentages of lymphocyte subpopulations.

EXERCISE AND NK CELLS

CHARACTERIZATION OF NK CELLS

NK cells are a heterogenous population of cells; by definition they are CD3$^-$ large granular lymphocytes that express characteristic NK cell markers such as CD16 and CD56; at least 50% of the cells also express CD2 (the sheep erythrocyte receptor). In addition, it has been shown that a subpopulation expresses the CD8 antigen at a density lower than that present on the CD16$^-$ T cells.[28] They mediate nonmajor histocompatibility complex (MHC)-restricted cytotoxicity and offer potential resistance to viral infections.[29] They also mediate cytotoxic activity against some malignant cells.[28] The cytotoxic activity of NK cells is enhanced by interferon (IFN)-α[30] and interleukin (IL)-2,[31] whereas certain prostaglandins[32] and immune complexes[33] downregulate the function of NK cells. The in vitro-generated lymphokine activated killer (LAK) cells show a broader range of non-MHC-restricted target cell killing.[34]

NK cells, therefore, are thought to play an important role in the first line of defense against acute and chronic virus infections and tumor spread.[35] It has often been said that NK cells are rapidly activated cells that offer resistance against viral infected and certain malignant cells until the specific T cell response has been developed.

The kinetics of NK cell activation during infection has been most systemically analyzed in mice infected with lymphocytic choriomeningitis virus. The NK cell response is augmented at early stages of infection, in parallel with the induction of IFN. This is followed by the virus-specific MHC-restricted cytotoxic T lymphocyte (CTL)-response. The augmented NK cell response that occurs after viral infection has been ascribed to two phenomena: (1) the activation of NK cells to a higher state of cytotoxicity; and (2) the proliferation of NK cells, which results in an increase in the number of NK cells.[36]

Studies in various stress models[11,37-41] show that high numbers of NK cells are recruited to the circulation within a few minutes after the onset of the stress and that NK cells are more sensitive to stress stimuli than any other subpopulations.[41] Results from the area of stress-immunology thus indicate that the rapidly increasing NK cell response in relation to infections probably also includes immediate recruitment of NK cells to the circulation and the site of infection.

THE PHENOTYPE OF NK CELLS DURING EXERCISE

Exercise of various types, durations and intensities causes recruitment to the blood of cells expressing characteristic NK cell markers, such as CD16 and CD56 (Table 2.1).[2,4,5,9-12,15,17,20,23-27,37,42-57]

An experiment was performed in our laboratory to characterize the phenotypes of NK cells recruited to the blood during exercise. Blood samples were collected before, at the end of 60 minutes of bicycle exercise at 75% of VO_2max as well as 2 hours and 4 hours after work.[58] Flow cytometric analysis identified cells expressing CD16 and CD56 alone or together with CD4, CD3 and CD8 as well as cells coexpressing CD16 and CD56. The %CD16$^+$ cells increased from 6-21%, the %CD16$^+$/CD8$^+$ cells increased from 2-6% and the %CD16$^+$/CD56$^+$ cells increased from 2-6%; in addition, the CD16$^+$/CD56$^+$ cells increased from 6-13% during exercise. The %CD16$^+$ cells coexpressing CD4 and CD3 did not change in relation to exercise. The %CD56$^+$ cells increased from 18-26% during exercise, whereas %CD56$^+$ cells coexpressing CD4, CD8 and CD3 did not change during exercise. It was concluded that the increase in NK cells during exercise was due to an increase in cells expressing either CD16 alone or in combination with CD8 or CD56, whereas there was no increase in the fraction of cells expressing CD56 alone or in combination with other cell markers.[58]

It is a general opinion that the majority of human NK cell activity is mediated by the CD16$^+$, CD56$^+$ and CD16$^+$CD56$^+$ cells.[28] In a recent investigation,[59] by the use of a large study material, Pearson's correlation analysis revealed that the NK cell activity was correlated with the percentages of CD16$^+$, CD56$^+$ and CD16$^+$/CD56$^+$ cells, but not to the CD16$^+$/CD8$^+$ cell subgroup. However, through linear multiple regression it was concluded that in controls the percentage of CD16$^+$ cells was the only parameter tested with any significant effect on NK cell activity.[59] Therefore, the finding that the NK cell pool during exercise differs from the NK cell pool before and after exercise mainly by an increased number of $CD16^+/CD56^-$ cells indicates the most active NK cells are recruited to the blood in response to exercise.

NK Cell Function During Exercise

Since the concentration of NK cells increases more than any other subpopulation of the lymphocytes, this means that the NK cell percentage of BMNC increases. Using an in vitro assay measuring the NK cell activity (lysis per fixed number of BMNC), the NK cell lysis increases as a consequence of increased proportion of cells mediating non-MHC-restricted cytotoxicity. During exercise the NK cell activity on a per NK cell basis does not change in some exercise models[20,53] but is reduced in relation to very intense exercise.[55]

In an early publication,[23] it was shown that NK cells with a high IL-2 response capacity were recruited to the blood during bicycle exercise. When BMNC were preincubated with IFN-α, IL-2 or indomethacin, a significant increase in the NK cell activity was registered at all the time points studied. During exercise the IL-2-enhanced NK cell activity increased significantly more than the IFN-α-enhanced NK cell activity (Fig. 2.3). When BMNC were incubated with IL-2 for more than 3 days to generate LAK cells, the LAK cell activity of cells from blood sampled at the end of the exercise period was significantly increased.[12] These data support the early findings[23] that during exercise NK cells with a high IL-2 response capacity is recruited to the blood.

NK Cell Function After Exercise

Following intense exercise of long duration, the concentration of NK cells declines below prevalues. Furthermore, the NK cell activity (lysis per fixed number of BMNC) decreases. The NK cell concentration and the NK cell activity are maximally suppressed 2-4 hours after exercise.

The percentage of NK cells has been found to be either unchanged compared to prevalues[60] or suppressed below prevalues.[24] In accordance with these controversial findings, the postexercise

Table 2.1. The effect of acute exercise on human NK cell activity, concentration and % CD16⁺ cells

Exercise Protocol	Lymphocyte B	Lymphocyte D	Lymphocyte A	CD16⁺ Con. B	CD16⁺ Con. D	CD16⁺ Con. A	CD16⁺ % B	CD16⁺ % D	CD16⁺ % A	NK Activity B	NK Activity D	NK Activity A	Notes
Brahmi[2] 1985 Cyc. exh. untr							58	0		31	59*	28*	Va=mean. Ch. % of prevalue E/T 20:1. D:IA
Brahmi[2] 1985 Cyc. exh. untr.							58	0		34	45*	28*	Va=mean. Ch. % of prevalue E/T 20:1. D:IA
Deuster[27] 1988 Treadmill to exh.	2.1	4.5*	1.3*	0.2	0.9*	0.1	8	16*	5				Va=mean. D:IA, A: 1 h
Edwards[26] 1984 Run 5 min	1.0	2.0			0.1	0.7				30	65*		Va=mean. E/T 20:1 D:IA
Espersen[42] 1990 Run 5 km	1.9	3.6*	1.1*				14	24*	15				Va=median. D:IA
Field[4] 1991 Cyc. exh. 12.9 m, Ex1	1.6	3.7*	1.0*	0.1	1.0*	0.1	10	25*	8	17	56*	20	Va=mean. D: at exh. A:1h, E/T 20:1
Field[4] 1991 Cyc. exh. 13.2 m, Ex2		3.1*	1.1*		0.9*	0.1							Ex2 1 h after Ex1. D: at exh. A:1 h, E/TVa=mean.20:1
Fry[5,6] 1992 Run 3 m exh	1.0	5.7*	1.0	0.5	2.0*	0.2	20	37*	15				Va=mean. D:IA CD16=CD56
Fry[5,6] 1992 Run 1 m 30%	2.5	1.9					8	8					Va=mean. D:<5 m pex. CD16=CD56
Fry[5,6] 1992 Run 1 m 60%	2.5	2.0					8	12					Va=mean. D:<5 m pex. CD16=CD56
Fry[5,6] 1992 Run 1 m 90%	2.5	2.6					8	21					Va=mean. D:<5 m pex. CD16=CD56
Fry[5,6] 1992 Run 1 m 120%	2.5	6.0*					8	30*					Va=mean. D:<5 m pex. CD16=CD56
Gabriel[43] 1992 Cyc. exh. 84 m	1.5	2.3*		0.2	0.*6								Va=mean. D:IA
Gabriel[9] 1992 Cyc. 60s max	1.5	2.9*	1.1*	0.2	1.0*	0.1*							Va=mean. D:IA
Haq[44] 1993 Marathon postrace	2.7		2.1	0.5		0.2*	19		10*				Va=mean A:10-15m

Table 2.1. The effect of acute exercise on human NK cell activity, concentration and % CD16⁺ cells (continued)

	Lymphocyte			CD16+ Con.			CD16+ %			NK Activity			Notes
Exercise Protocol	**B**	**D**	**A**	**B**	**D**	**A**	**B**	**D**	**A**	**B**	**D**	**A**	
Hoffmann 1990 Goetz[10] Cyc. 1 h 65%max Day1	1.9	2.7*		0.2	0.5*		11	18*					Va=mean D: 3 m pex.
Hoffmann 1990 Goetz[10] Cyc. 1 h 65%max Day2	1.7	2.4*		0.2	0.5*		10	18*					Va=mean D: 3 m pex.
Hoffmann 1990 Goetz[10] Cyc. 1 h 65%max Day3	1.6	1.8*		0.2	0.4*		13	17*					Va=mean D: 3 m pex.
Kappel[11] 1991 Cyc. 1 h 75%max	2.3	4.7*	1.3*	1.0	2.3	1.2	24	46*	16*				Va=mean. E/T 50:1
Klokker[37] 1995 Cyc. 50% VO_2max				0.2	0.5*		21	31*		32	45*		Va=mean E/T 50:1, D: IA
Nielsen[54] 1996 Rowing 6 m a-o	1.4	4.2*	1.0*	0.2	1.5*	0.2	12	32*	10	25	47	24	Va=mean E/T 100:1, A:2 h
Nielsen[55] 1996 Rowing 6 m rep a-o	1.2	5.1*	1.5*	0.1	1.2*	0.1	5	18*	5	10	40*	10	Va=mean D:last of six bouts
Nieman[45] 1991 Walk 1 h 60%max	1.9	2.3*	1.8	0.3	0.5*	0.2*							Va=mean A:1.5 h
Nieman[17] 1992 Cyc. 30 s max	2.5	3.2*	1.6*	0.4	1.0*	0.2*							Va=mean D:3 m pex. A:1 h
Nieman[20] 1993 Run 45 m moderate	2.3	2.5	1.5				14	19*	10*	50	70	30	Va=mean NK:LU,D:IA,A:1 h
Nieman[20] 1993 Run 45 m high	2.3	4.0*	1.3*				18	27*	8*	55	100*	30	Va=mean NK:LU,D:IA,A:1 h
Nieman[57] 1995 Leg squat exh.	2.2	4.3*	1.4*	0.5	1.6*	0.3*				34	35*	13*	Va=mean NK:LU,D:IA,A:2 h
Palmø[53] 1995 One leg. ec. ex.	1.7	2.2*	1.4*				9	18*	8	28	47*	24	Va=mean E/T 50:1,A:4 h
Pedersen[24] 1990 Cyc. 1 h 75%VO2max	2.2	5.1*	1.1*				11	24*	12	30	49*	20*	Va=median. E/T 50:1
Pedersen[23] 1988 Cyc. 1 h 75%VO_2max	2.4	5.4*	1.8*				12	30*	12	34	50*	20*	Va=median. E/T 50:1
Rhind[56] 1994 Cyc. exh. untr.			2.3			0.2							Va=mean A:one week
Rhind[56] 1994 Cyc. exh. tr.			1.9			0.3							Va=mean A:one week
Shinkai[25] 1992 Cyc. 1 h 75%VO_2max	1.8	2.6*	1.1*	2.5	6.5*	0.6*	13	25*	6*	100	160	55	Va=mean A:60m
Targan[46] 1981 Cyc. 5 m 25 mph											32	55*	Va=mean D:5 m pex. E/T 20:1

Table continues on following page.

Table 2.1. The effect of acute exercise on human NK cell activity, concentration and % CD16⁺ cells (continued)

Exercise Protocol	Lymphocyte			CD16⁺ Con.			CD16⁺ %			NK Activity			Notes
	B	D	A	B	D	A	B	D	A	B	D	A	
Tvede[15] 1989 Cyc. 1 h 75%VO_2max	2.1	4.3*	1.1*	0.3	1.2*	0.1*	20	24*	11				Va=median
Tvede[12] 1993 Cyc. 1 h 25%VO_2max		10	-20					65*	-10*		67*	-13*	Va=median. E/T 100:1. Changes in % of prevalue
Tvede[12] 1993 Cyc. 1 h 50%VO_2max		40*	-35*					100*	-25*		87*	-11*	Va=median. E/T 100:1. Changes in % of prevalue
Tvede[12] 1993 Cyc. 1 h 75%VO_2max		125*	-23*					90*	-5*		75*	–25*	Va=median. E/T 100:1. Changes in % of prevalue
Ullum[21] 1994 Cyc. 1 h 75%VO_2max	2.0	3.2	1.2				12	22*	13	25	45*	25	Va=mean E/T 50:1, A:2 h

A, after; B, before (rest); CD, cell designation; conc, concentration; cyc, cycling; D, during; ec, eccentric; E/T, effector cell: target cell ratio; Ex, exercise; exh, exhaustion; D:IA, immediate after LU, lytic units; m, minutes; max, maximal; mph, miles per hour; pex, postexercise; s, seconds; tr, trained; untr, untrained; Va, value; VO_2max, maximal oxygen uptake.
Values "after" were measured two hours post-exercise; if different *Notes* describe measure points. Cell concentrations are given as cells x 10^9 l-1 or cells x 10^6 ml-1.
*, indicate significant value compared to rest ($P < 0.05$).

suppression of the NK cell activity has been ascribed to a decreased proportion of NK cells among BMNC. Furthermore, it has also been shown that the NK cell activity was not suppressed on a per NK cell basis following moderate exercise, but that the NK cell activity on a "per cell" basis was elevated postexercise.[20]

In other studies, it was suggested that the suppressed NK cell activity was due to downregulation of the NK cell activity by prostaglandins.[24] Previous reports have shown that the NK cell activity is downregulated by prostaglandins E1, E2 and D2.[61,62] In vitro indomethacin enhanced the NK cell activity of BMNC, but not of monocyte-depleted effector cells, indicating that the effect of indomethacin was due to inhibition of prostaglandins produced by monocytes.[63] The NK cell activity was also downregulated by the supernatants from autologous stimulated polymorphonuclear

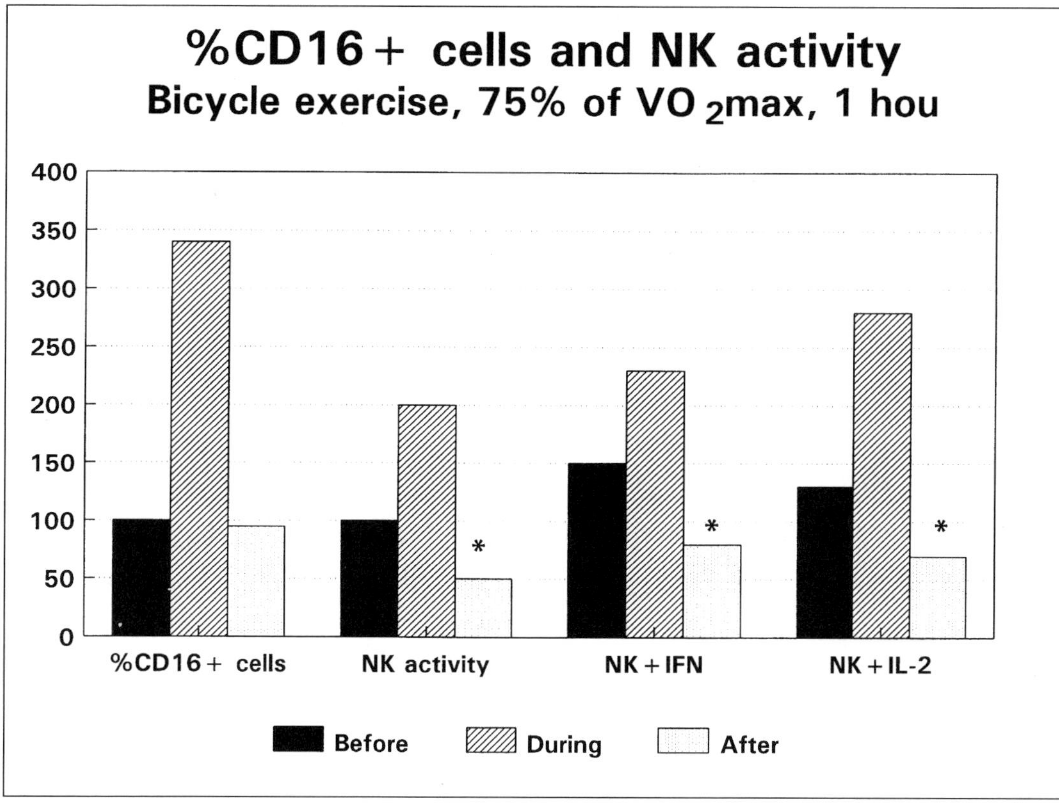

*Fig. 2.3. Percent CD16⁺ natural killer (NK) cells, unstimulated, interferon (IFN)-α and interleukin-2 (IL-2)-stimulated NK cell activity against K562 target cells before, during and after 60 minutes of bicycle exercise at 75% of VO_2max. * denotes significant difference from prevalues. Results are adapted from Pedersen et al.[23]*

neutrophils.[64] The presence of indomethacin in the in vitro mixture, or given orally to donors, partially or completely abolished the inhibitory effects of activated polymorphonuclear neutrophils.[64]

Two hours after bicycle exercise, the percentage of NK cells ($CD16^+$ cells) had returned to prevalues, but the NK cell activity was suppressed and the concentration of monocytes and neutrophils increased during the 2 hours postexercise period. The in vitro release of prostaglandin E_2 (PGE_2) from BMNC was increased and the neutrophil chemiluminescence response was also increased. The latter response is associated with PGE_2 production by neutrophils.

Indomethacin, whether administered in vitro or in vivo, fully restored the suppressed postexercise NK cell activity. Finally, the NK cell activity of monocyte-depleted BMNC did not decrease below basal levels after exercise.[24] This study indicates that prostaglandins released from monocytes and neutrophils are involved in the postexercise suppression of NK cells (Fig. 2.4). However, in a study by Nieman et al,[65] indomethacin in vitro did not abolish postexercise suppression of indomethacin. In the latter study, the NK cell percentage dropped postexercise and the NK cell activity was not found to be inhibited on a per NK cell basis. It is possible that the divergent findings reflect that a cycle model was used in our study[24] and a running model was used in the study by Nieman et al.[65]

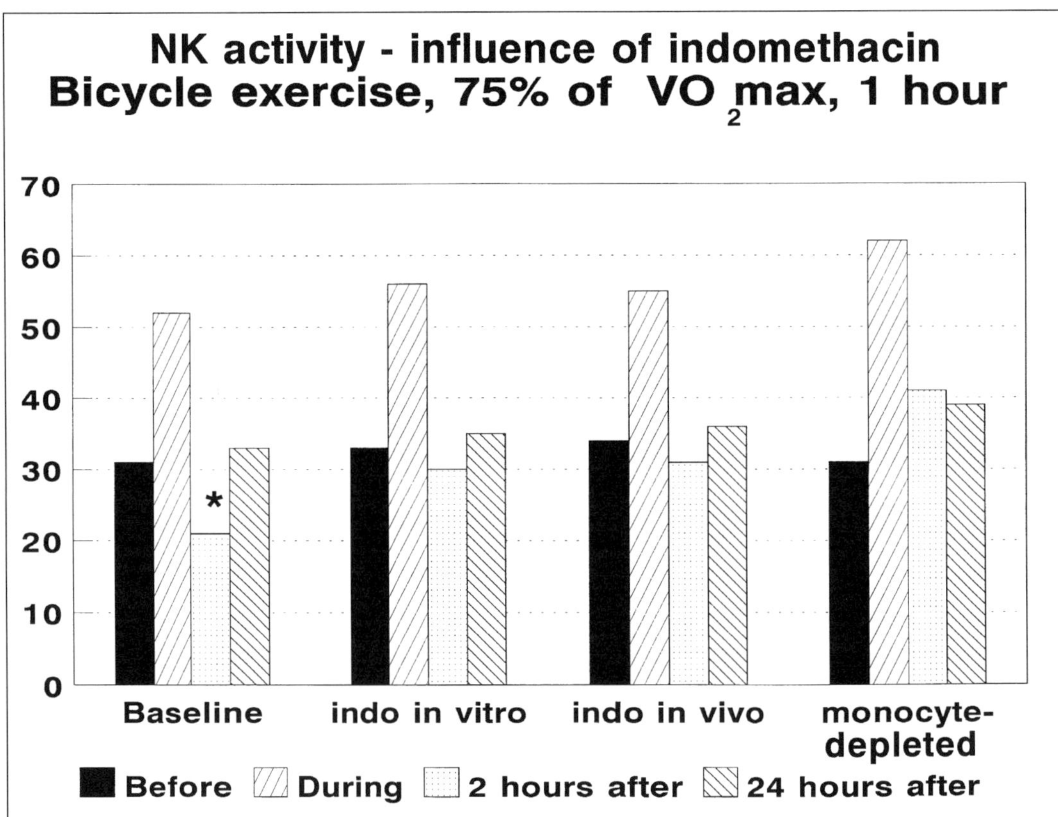

*Fig. 2.4. Natural killer (NK) cell activity against K562 target cells before, during and after 60 minutes of bicycle exercise at 75% of VO_2max. The effect of indomethacin (1 µg/ml) in vitro on NK cell activity is shown. NK cell activity in relation to exercise in untreated individuals and in same individuals treated with indomethacin for 2 days. The effect of monocyte-depletion on NK cell activity of blood mononuclear cells (BMNC). * denotes significant difference from prevalues. Results are adapted from Pedersen et al.[24]*

NK Cells at Exercise of Different Duration and Intensity

The available data on human NK cells and NK cell activity in relation to an acute bout of exercise are summarized in Table 2.1. The NK cells have been studied in various models; including laboratory and field studies; studies on running, cycling and rowing; studies on concentric, eccentric or combined concentric and eccentric exercise; and exercise lasting from a few minutes to several hours.[2,4,5,9-12,15,17,20,23-27,37,42-53,66-68]

In general, the NK cell activity is increased when measured immediately after or during both moderate and intense exercise of a few minutes. The intensity, more than the duration of exercise, is responsible for the degree of increment in the number of NK cells. If the exercise has lasted for a long period and has been very intense (e.g., a triathlon race), only a modest increase in NK cells are found postexercise.[69]

The NK cell count and the NK cell activity is suppressed only following intense exercise of a certain duration, and at least 1 hour seems to be a critical duration of exercise in terms of postexercise suppression of natural immunity. Initial fitness level or sex do not influence the magnitude of exercise-induced changes in NK cells.[2]

Based on the available data a model on exercise, duration and intensity is suggested. NK cells and other lymphocytes are recruited from a pool. This pool may be located in various organs such as the spleen, the lungs, the bone marrow and the lymph nodes. The number of cells that enter the circulation are determined by the intensity of the stimulus. If it has been a long lasting and very intense stimulus the total concentration of lymphocytes decline. This may in part be because there are no more mature cells to recruit, or it may be ascribed to a redistribution of lymphocytes from the circulation to organs. However, a recent animal study failed to show accumulation of lymphocytes in skeletal muscles after exercise.[70]

Whether or not the "open window" in the immune system occurs is therefore dependent on a combination of intensity and duration. It remains to be shown whether the degree of muscle damage also play a role, e.g., if lymphopenia occurs earlier during running exercise (concentric and eccentric exercise) than during cycling (concentric exercise), at the same VO_2.

EXERCISE AND LYMPHOCYTE PROLIFERATION

To function in adaptive immunity, rare antigen-specific lymphocytes must proliferate extensively before they differentiate into functional effector cells, in order to generate sufficient numbers of effector cells of a particular specificity. Therefore, the assessment of lymphocyte function in relation to exercise has involved the analysis of induced lymphocyte proliferation as a central issue. It is difficult to study the proliferation of normal lymphocytes in response to specific antigens because only a minor proportion of cells will be stimulated to divide. However, most studies on lymphocyte proliferation have used polyclonal mitogens, which induce many or all lymphocytes of a given type to proliferate. Although the polyclonal mitogens likely do not act directly on the antigen-specific receptors of lymphocytes, they seem to trigger the same growth response mechanisms as antigens. Lymphocytes normally exist as resting cells in the G0 phase of the cell cycle. When stimulated with polyclonal antigens, they rapidly enter G1 and progress through the cell cycle. This process can be monitored by using the fluorescence activated cell sorter (FACS) to analyze their DNA or RNA content. However, most studies of lymphocyte proliferation analyze the incorporation of ^{3}H-thymidine into the DNA cells as a sign of cell growth.[71]

It appears from Table 2.2 that highly variable results on lymphocyte proliferation in humans have been found. However, most studies in humans show that the phytohemagglutinin (PHA) and concanavalian A (ConA) responses decline during exercise, and this has also been a consistent finding in animal studies.[4,5,12,18,21,25,57,72-79]

Tvede et al[15] studied the proliferative response and distribution of BMNC subpopulations in relation to concentric bicycle exercise at 75% of VO_2max for 1 hour. In accordance with many other studies, the PHA response declined, the %$CD4^+$ cells declined and the %$CD16^+$ cells increased during exercise. In order to determine whether a single subpopulation of BMNC was responsible for the suppressed PHA proliferative response during work, BMNC were cultured in the presence of PHA, pulsed with ^{3}H-thymidine, followed by FACS-sorting into $CD4^+$ and $CD8^+$ subgroups.

The proliferative response per fixed number of BMNC did not change during or after bicycle exercise. However, the proliferative contribution of the $CD4^+$ subgroup (percentage of total ^{3}H-thymidine incorporation) declined during bicycle exercise due to the declined proportion of $CD4^+$ cells (Fig. 2.5).

The ability of BMNC to proliferate in response to a physiological dose of IL-2 may be a more relevant test of cellular activation than the use of nonspecific mitogens. Activation of T-lymphocytes leads to production of the growth factor IL-2[80] and to the expression of the low affinity IL-2 receptor (IL-2R).[81] It is known that the IL-2 proliferative signal is mediated by

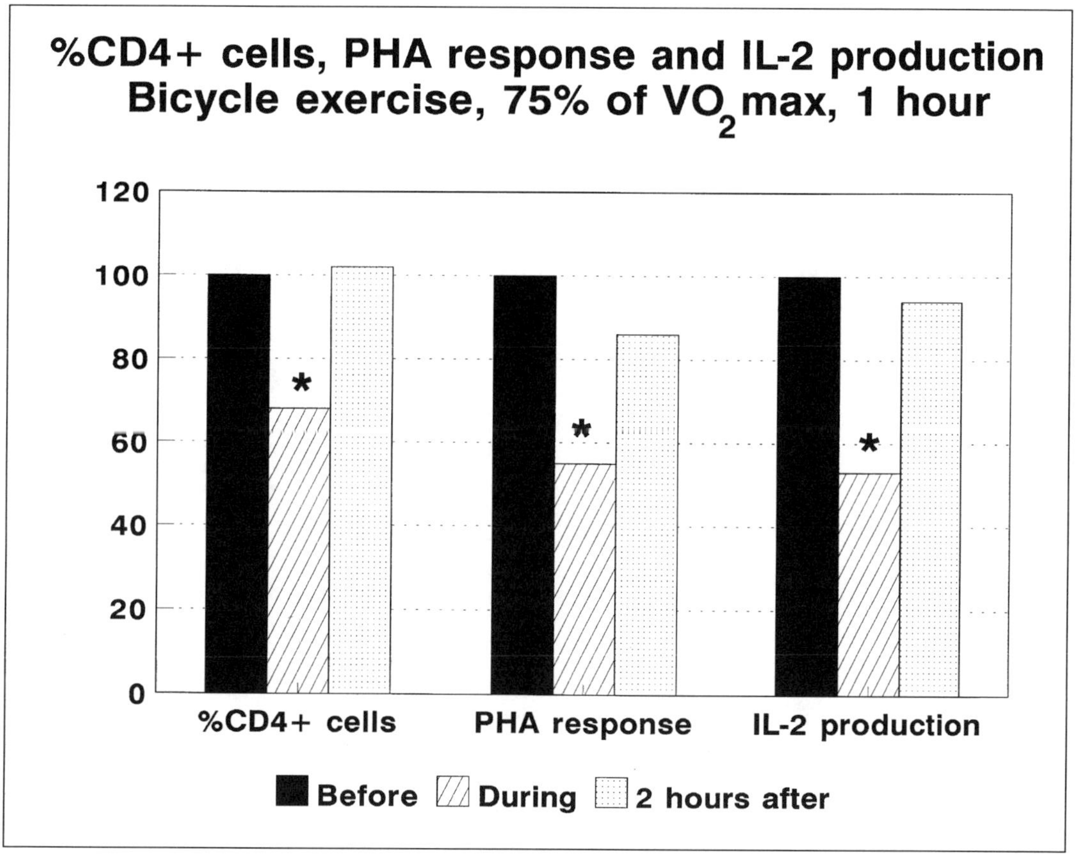

*Fig. 2.5. The %$CD4^+$ cells. The proliferative response following stimulation with phytohemagglutinin (PHA) and the production of interleukin (IL)-2 from PHA-stimulated BMNC. The decreased PHA-response was due to a relative fall in $CD4^+$ cells. * denotes significant difference from prevalues. Results are partly adapted from Tvede et al.[15]*

Table 2.2. The effect of acute exercise on human lymphocyte proliferative response

Ref.	Exercise	N	Subj.	P.time h/Th	Stim.	Effect D	Effect A1	Effect A2	Notes A1: 10m A
Edwards[26] *1984*	Running stairs, 5 m	7	ND	96/?	ConA;		–		–
Eskola[74] *1978*	Marathon best: 2.5 h	8	ND	72/18	ConA; 100		↓	↓	
				–	PHA; 100		↓	↓	A1: 30 m
				96/18	PPD; 100,1		↓	↓	A2: 3 h
Espersen[42] *1991*	Running 5 km, 15-18 m	11	V^K:55	72/?	ConA; 62.5,25	–	↑	–	
				–	PHA; 500,100,20	–	↑	–	A1: 2 h
					PWM; 50	–	↑	–	A2: 24 h
Field[4] *1991*	Cycling to exh. 13 m	12	V:3.5	96/18	ConA; 100	–	–		
					PHA; 10	↓	↓		
					PMA; 20	↓	↓		
					PWM; 1	↓	–		A1: 1 h
Fry[6] *1992a*	Treadmill	7							
	rep. ex. 3 m +			72/24	ConA; 3.1	↓	–		A1: 0.5+1 h
	int: 0-120% 5-20 km h^{-1}			72/24	ConA; 3.1	↓			D:5 m A 120%
Fry[6] *1992b*	Treadmill rep. 3 m pro.	7	V:4.6	72/24	ConA; 3.1	↓	–		D:3-5 m A
				–	PHA; 3.1	↓	–		A1:2,4, 8,24 h
MacNeil[77] *1991*	Cycling 30-120 m 30-75%	32	LV:45	72/8	ConA; 2.5	–	↓	–	D:3m A
			MV:55	–	–	↓	↓	↓	A1:0.5,2 h
			HV:63	–	–	–	–	–	A2:24 h
Nehlsen[18] *1991*	Walking 45 m 59%	12	V^K:26	84/12	ConA; 5	–	–	–	D;IA;A
					PHA; 5	–	↓	–	1:1.5+3 h A2:5+23 h

Nielsen[55] *1996*	Rowing "all-out" 6 m	7	V:	72/24	IL2; 20	–	–		
				–	PHA; 3	–	–		
				–	PPD; 10	–	–		
Nieman[57]	Leg squat 3 m 1 rep. pr. 6 s	10	V^K:44	76/4	ConA; 20	–	–		D:IA *1995* A1: 2 h
Shinkai[25] *1992*	Cycling 60 m 60%	21	V^K:41	72/6	PHA; 40	↓	–	–	A1:0.5,1 h
				–	PWM; 20	↓	↑	–	A2:2 h
Smith[67] *1993*	Running 6.6 km	25	ND	96/6	ConA; 5,10	–	–	–	A1:30m,1 h
				–	PHA;5,10	↓	↓	–	A2:2,4,6 h
				–	PWM;5,10	↓	–	–	
Tvede[15] *1989*	Cycling 60 m 75%	16		72/24	PHA; 3	↓	–	–	A1:2 h
				–	PPD; 10	–	–	–	A2:24 h
Tvede[14] *1994*	Cycling 60 m 75%	8	V^K:55	72/24	IL2; 20	↑	↑		A1:2 h
				–	PHA; 3	↓	–		
				–	PPD; 10	–	–		
Tvede[14] *1994*	Cycling 60 m 25-75%	6	V^K:56	72/24	IL2; 20	↑	–		A1:2 h,IL2↑: 50+75%
				–	PHA; 3	↓	–		D, 25%A
				–	PPD; 10	–	–		PHA↓:75%
Ullum[21] *1994*	Cycling 60 m 75%	8	V^K:47	72/24	IL2; 20	–	–		A1:2 h
				–	PHA; 3	–	–		
				–	PPD; 10	–	–		
Verde[68] *1992*	Treadmill 30 m 80%	10	V^K:65	72/24	ConA; 1,2,4	–	↑		D:5 m A;
				–	PHA; 10,15,20	↓	–		A1:30 m

A, after; D, during; ConA, concanavalin A; exh, exhaustion; h, hours; IA, immediately after; int, different intensities; IL2, interleukin-2; m, minutes; N, number of subjects; ND, subjects are not desribed; nm, near maximal; PHA, phytohemagglutinin; PPD, purified protein derivative of tuberculin; PWM, pokeweed mitogen; P.time, time of proliferation; s, seconds; sp, speed; stim, agents of stimulation; V, maximal oxygen uptake; V^K, maximal oxygen uptake related to body weight. Figures following *stim.* describes concentration of each used. Amount of stim. are either final of start concentration. ConA, PHA, PPD and PWM are given in μg ml^{-1} and IL-2 in U ml^{-1}.

the binding and internalization of the high affinity IL-2R,[82] and this is why the IL-2 mitogenic effect on lymphocytes correlates to the expression of high affinity IL-2R.

During exercise, an increased proliferative response to IL-2 was found despite unchanged IL-2R expression. The most IL-2 responsive cells among the subpopulations were found to be the $CD16^+$ NK cells. The contribution of the $CD16^+$ cells increased during exercise and FACS-sorting revealed that the proliferative response per cell did not change in relation to exercise. Therefore, the increase in IL-2 response during physical activity reflects changes in cell composition and is not a consequence of cellular activation (Tvede et al, unpublished data).

The finding that the PHA- and ConA-induced lymphocyte proliferative responses decline during exercise has incorrectly been called "immunosuppression." However, it is important to bear in mind that during exercise more lymphocytes are recruited to the blood and on a per cell basis, the lymphocyte proliferative response is not suppressed. Thus, the suppressed PHA- and conA-responses during exercise simply reflect that the NK cells increase more than the T cells during exercise. Following exercise, the total lymphocyte concentration declines and the proliferative response is either unchanged or not different from prevalues. As a consequence the total in vivo lymphocyte function in the blood is suppressed after exercise.

EXERCISE AND ANTIBODY PRODUCTION

The secretory immune system of mucosal tissues such as the upper respiratory tract is considered to be the first barrier to colonization by pathogenic microorganisms causing upper respiratory tract infections.[83-85] Although IgA constitutes only 10-15% of the total immunoglobulin in serum, it is the predominant immunoglobulin class in mucosal secretions, and the level of IgA in mucosal fluids correlates more closely with resistance to upper respiratory tract infections than serum antibodies.[86]

Tomasi et al[87] reported suppressed levels of the salivary IgA in cross-country skiers after a race. This finding was confirmed by a 70% decrease in salivary IgA for several hours after 2 hours of intense ergometer cycling.[88] Decreased salivary IgA was found after swimming,[89] in addition salivary IgA was low for several hours after marathon running[90] and incremental treadmill running to exhaustion.[91] Submaximal exercise of VO_2max had no effect on salivary IgA.[92,93]

In order to study the mechanism behind the suppression of immunoglobulins, a plaque forming cell assay has been used. This assay allows an identification of the individual immunoglobulin-secreting cells of blood. Stimulation of cells with pokeweed mitogen, IL-2 and Epstein-Barr virus resulted in significantly decreased numbers of IgG, IgA and IgM-secreting blood cells during exercise, as well as 2 hours postexercise. Recovery occurred after 1 day (Fig. 2.6).

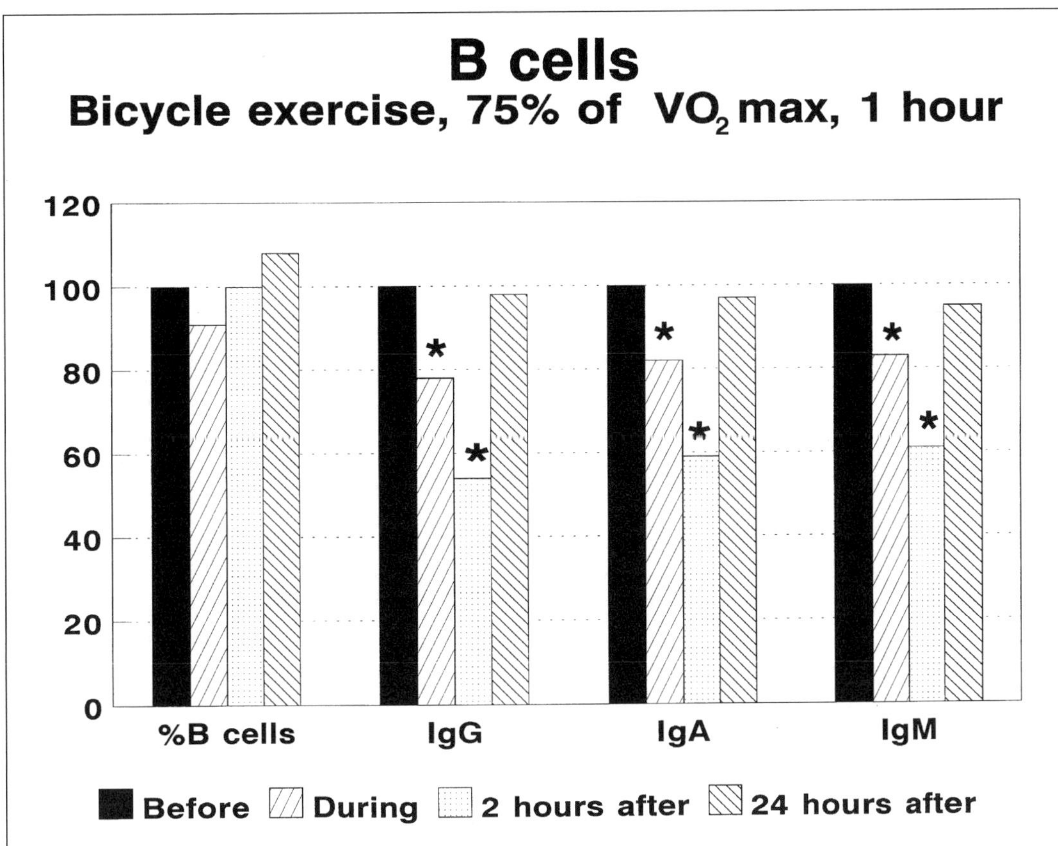

*Fig. 2.6. The percentages of CD19⁺ B cells, the IgG, IgM and IgA plaque forming cells (PFC) responses of poke weed mitogen (PWM)-stimulated blood mononuclear cells (BMNC) isolated before, during, 2 and 4 hours postexercise. * denotes significant difference from prevalues. Results are adapted from Tvede et al.[22]*

The percentage of B cells among BMNC does not change in relation to exercise, suggesting that the suppression of immunoglobulin-secreting cells is not due to changes in numbers of B cells. Purified B cells produce plaques only after stimulation with Epstein-Barr virus and in these cultures no exercise-induced suppression was found. The addition of indomethacin to IL-2 stimulated cultures of blood mononuclear cells partly reversed the postexercise suppressed B cell function.

Therefore, it was concluded that the exercise-induced suppression of the plaque forming cell response was partly mediated by monocytes.[22]

CELLULAR ACTIVATION IN RESPONSE TO EXERCISE

Exercise induces numerous changes in the immune system, but it is highly debated whether these changes reflect activation of the immune system or changed composition of lymphocyte subpopulations influencing the functional in vitro assays. Certainly, many of the exercise-induced changes that have been described can be ascribed to changes in the composition of BMNC. For example, the increased NK cell activity during exercise is due to an increased percentage of NK cells, the decreased PHA response is due to the decreased fraction of the $CD4^+$ cells, the increased IL-2-induced proliferation is due to an increased fraction of $CD16^+$ cells and the increased in vitro production of IL-1 from endotoxin-stimulated BMNC is due to increased percentage of monocytes.

However, the increased levels of cytokines in plasma following intense exercise cannot be ascribed to redistribution of monocytes.[42,94-98] Tilz et al[99] found increased plasma concentrations of soluble IL-2R, CD8, intercellular adhesion molecule 1 (ICAM1), CD23, tumor necrosis factor-α-receptor (TNF-αR) and neopterin in 18 individuals during, or after, long-duration exercise. These results suggest that there is some immune system activation during intense exercise of long duration. However, in another study the levels of colony-stimulating factor and neopterin remained unchanged after concentric exercise.[100] Gabriel et al[101] found increased $CD45RA^+$-$45RO^+$ cells after endurance exercise and suggested that this might reflect activation of the T cells.

Dufaux et al[85,102] suggested that prolonged severe physical exercise was associated with an initial increase and delayed decrease in circulating immune complexes. However, the changes were, although statistically significant, quantitatively small and the values were only occasionally above the upper limit. Studies by Thomsen et al[103] and Simpson et al[104] do not indicate these changes. The lack of increased concentrations of immune complexes and also the lack of occurrence of C3c and C3d indicate that immune complex-induced complement activation does not occur during concentric exercise.[103] Furthermore, the levels of complement receptor type one (CR1) on erythrocytes does not change in relation to concentric exercise, neither in healthy subjects nor in patients with rheumatoid arthritis.[103]

Camus et al[105] studied the effects of exercise on the plasma levels of myeloperoxidase and C5a, taken as specific markers of polymorphonuclear neutrophil and complement activation, respectively. The plasma levels of myeloperoxidase and C5a increased during exercise. The similar time course of changes in myeloperoxidase and C5a, and the highly significant relationship between these two variables, lend some support to the hypothesis that complement activation contributes to postexercise neutrocytosis in eccentric exercise.

The disparity between the studies[85,102-105] may be explained by the fact that only exercise of long duration or exercise involving an eccentric component cause activation of the complement cascade. In support of this hypothesis, Camus et al[106] showed that downhill running, but not uphill walking induced increased plasma levels of myeloperoxidase and elastase. Thus, in general, the studies mentioned above suggest that eccentric but not concentric exercise induces activation of the immune system.

EXERCISE AND IN VIVO IMMUNOLOGICAL METHODS

Several studies have investigated the immune system in relation to exercise, employing in vitro immunological methods. Only a few studies have monitored the immune system in relation to exercise using in vivo immunological methods. Bruunsgaard et al[107] investigated whether an in vivo impairment of cell-mediated immunity and specific antibody production could be demonstrated after intense exercise of long duration (triathlon race).

The cellular immune system was evaluated as the skin test response to seven recall antigens while the humoral immune system was evaluated as the antibody response to pneumococcal polysaccharide vaccine, which is generally considered to be T cell independent, and two toxoids (tetanus and diphtheria) that are dependent on T cells.

The skin test response was significantly suppressed in the group who performed a triathlon race compared to triathlete controls and untrained controls, who did not participate in the triathlon. No differences in specific antibody titers were found between the groups. The latter is in accordance with the findings by Eskola et al.[74]

Thus, in vivo cell-mediated immunity was impaired in the first days after prolonged, high intensity exercise, whereas there was no impairment of the in vivo antibody production measured 2 weeks after vaccination. The explanation of this may be that primarily unspecific immunity is influenced by exercise, whereas the specificity of the immune system is not altered. Alternatively, the time factor may be taken into consideration, thus during the 2 week period the immune system may have had time to regenerate.

NEUTROPHIL FUNCTION

Neutrophils represent 50-60% of the total circulating leukocyte pool. They are considered to be part of the innate immune system and are essential for host defense. However, they are also involved in the pathology of various inflammatory conditions. Therefore, neutrophils can be considered to be a double-edged sword, as suggested by Smith.[108]

One of the more pronounced features of physical activity on immune parameters is the prolonged neutrocytosis following acute longterm exercise.[1] Short bouts of vigorous exercise lasting from approximately 10 seconds to 0.5 hour (e.g., sprinting, rowing or gymnastics), sustained strenuous exercise lasting a few hours (e.g., marathon races), or intermittent vigorous exercise (e.g., American football or soccer), can all induce in the participants an immediate leukocytosis.[1] At the end of short term exercise lasting up to 0.5 hour the leukocyte count usually falls quickly, approaching its normal levels within 0.5 hour. After sustained exercise, lasting

2.5-3.5 hours, the leukocyte count returns slowly and is often elevated above preexercise levels at 24 hours. Whereas after intermittent exercise over 1.5 hours or sustained exercise of 1 hour, the leukocyte count continues to rise for 1-4 hours before falling slowly.[108-110]

There are a number of reports showing that exercise triggers a series of changes in the neutrophil population and may affect certain subpopulations differentially. Kurokawa et al[111] reported a fall in expression of L-selectin (CD62L) immediately after exercise followed by an increase during recovery, whereas there were no changes in CD11a or CD11b expression. Smith et al[112] showed increased expression of CD11b in response to exercise.

Regarding the function of neutrophils, exercise has both short- and long-term effects. The neutrophil response to infections, include adherence, chemotaxis, phagocytosis, oxidative burst, degranulation and microbial killing. In general, moderate exercise boosts neutrophil functions; including chemotaxis, phagocytosis and the oxidative burst; whereas extreme exercise suppresses these functions with the exception of chemotaxis and degranulation, which are not affected.[109,113-116]

In the study by Smith et al,[109] neutrophil killing capacity was enhanced for at least 6 hours following 1 hour of moderate ergometer cycle exercise. In another study, immediately following a 20 km race, neutrophils from runners were less able to ingest bacteria, an effect which lasted for 3 days.[113]

In a comparative study of male distance runners, triathletes and untrained controls, progressive exercise to exhaustion doubled neutrophil phagocytic capacity in samples taken up to 24 hours after exercise. Superoxide production in phorbol myristate acetate stimulated cells fell slightly immediately after exercise but then increased 1 hour later and remained elevated for 24 hours; there were significant changes in chemotactic capacity or random migration.[117] These results were confirmed by the same group in both trained and untrained individuals.[118] Phagocytic activity increased immediately after exercise but no changes in adherence or bactericidal activity were described in untrained individuals. However, decreased adherence and bactericidal activity, but no change in phagocytic activity, were found in elite cyclists.[119]

Prolonged impaired neutrophil function has also been reported in race horses following a single strenuous event.[120] Several studies have shown that exercise activates the release of neutrophil granule constituents into the circulation, indicating direct neutrophil activation in vivo. Elevated concentrations of neutrophil elastase have been detected in plasma after exercise.[106,121-124]

REPETITIVE BOUTS OF ACUTE EXERCISE

Little is known about the effects of repeated bouts of exercise. Hoffman-Goetz et al[10] studied the effect of repeated bouts of submaximal cycle ergometry exercise on changes in the percentage of BMNC subpopulations. Healthy volunteers exercised daily for 1 hour at 65% of VO_2max. The increase in percentage of NK cells to five repetitive bouts of cycling over 5 days was not different from that elicited by the first bout.[10]

Field et al[4] studied the effect of two bouts of exhaustive cycle ergometry exercise, each lasting 12.9 minutes and 13.2 minutes, respectively, and separated by 1 hour. A significant increase in total leukocytes (2-fold), neutrophils (1.9-fold) and lymphocytes (2.3-fold) occurred with the first exercise bout. The concentrations of leukocytes and neutrophils increased to the same level with both experiments, but the concentrations 1 hour after the second bout were higher than that 1 hour after the first bout of exercise. The concentration of lymphocytes increased less with the second bout compared to the first bout of exercise. One hour after the second bout, the lymphocyte concentration decreased below prevalues. This suppression was similar to that developed following the first bout of exercise.

Nielsen et al[54] investigated the effects on the immune system of 6 minutes "all-out" ergometer rowing over 2 days (two x three bouts) in elite male oarsmen. Compared to levels at rest, the first bout of exercise increased the concentration of leukocytes (2-fold), neutrocytes (2-fold), lymphocytes (2-fold); the BMNC subsets—$CD3^+$ (2-fold), $CD4^+$ (2-fold), $CD8^+$ (3-fold), $CD16^+$ (8-fold), $CD19^+$ (2-fold); and the NK cell activity (2-fold). During the last bout, even higher levels were noted for leukocytes (3-fold), neutrocytes (3-fold) and lymphocytes (4-fold); the BMNC subsets—

$CD4^+$ (3-fold), $CD8^+$ (5-fold), $CD16^+$ (13-fold), $CD19^+$ (5-fold); and NK cell activity (4-fold). During the recovery periods all values were at or above the level at rest, and elevated concentrations of leukocytes, neutrocytes, lymphocytes and NK cell activity were also noted on the day following the last bout.

The divergence between the studies by Hoffman-Goetz,[10] Field et al[4] and Nielsen et al[54] may reflect that enhancement of the immune system depends on the intensity of exercise. The results by Nielsen et al[54] show that intense exercise of short duration with large muscle groups does not induce immunosuppression, but provokes higher immune responses during repetitive bouts of exercise.

THE ROLE OF THE SPLEEN IN EXERCISE

The exercise-related neutrocytosis is thought to be due to movement of neutrophils from marginal pools located intravascularly and from extravascular storage pools. The role of the lung vasculature in neutrophilic granulocyte sequestration has been repeatedly demonstrated.[125]

Concerning lymphocytes the concept of margination is less clear. An effect of the spleen may contribute to the lymphocytosis. The spleen is the major storage pool of lymphocytes, and 2.5×10^{11} cells per day recirculate between the blood and the pulpa[126] and splenic sympathetic nerve activity reduces the splenic NK cell activity.[127] Thus, splenectomized subjects demonstrate a low lymphocyte count in response to injection of adrenaline and subjects without a spleen show less relative increase of lymphocytes during exercise (Nielsen et al, manuscript submitted for publication). The latter results were in contrast to the finding that the spleen does not play a role in exercise-leukocytosis.[129]

THE OPEN WINDOW HYPOTHESIS

In essence, the immune system is enhanced during moderate and severe exercise, and only intense long-duration exercise is followed by a suppressed concentration of lymphocytes, suppressed non-MHC-restricted cytotoxicity (NK and LAK cell activity) and decreased concentration of secretory IgA in mucosa. Thus, following intense long-duration exercise, the immune system is temporarily suppressed. This period has also been called the "open window" (Fig. 2.7).[58]

During the "open window," microbacterial agents, especially viruses, may invade the host and infections may be established. One reason for the increased susceptibility to infections seen in elite athletes could be that this window of opportunism for pathogens is longer and the degree of immunosuppression more pronounced. We hypothesize that severe immunodepression may occur if athletes do not allow the immune system to recover but initiate a new bout of exercise, while still immunodepressed.

It has recently been suggested that neutrophils serve as a last line of defense. During the "open window" immune suppression

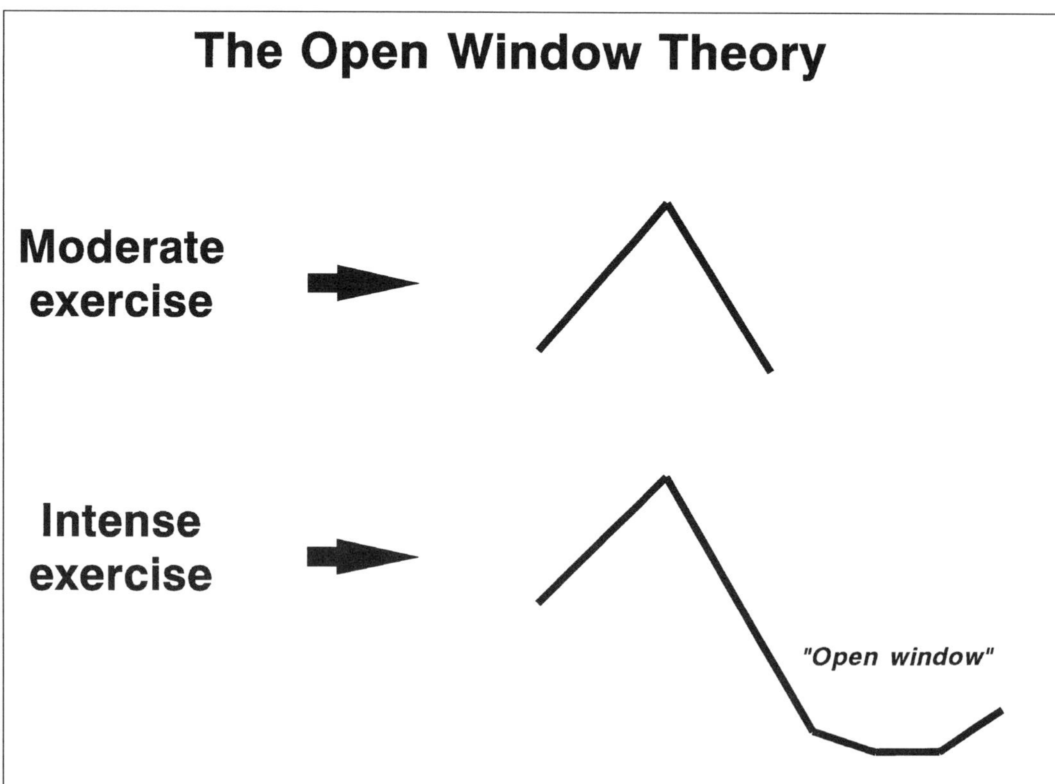

Fig. 2.7. Schematic presentation of the effects of moderate and intense exercise on the immune system. The model included the exercise effects of lymphocyte number, natural killer and lymphokine activated killer cell activities and antibody production. During moderate to severe exercise, the immune system is enhanced, but severe exercise is followed by a period of immunosuppression during which there is an "open window" of opportunity for pathogens. The model is adapted from Pedersen and Ullum[58] and Brines et al.[116]

of lymphoid cells, neutrophils are being mobilized to plug these gaps. The removal of this back-up system following extreme activity would be compatible with the increased frequency of upper respiratory tract infections in athletes.[116]

Several studies suggest that poststress immunosuppression is correlated to increased frequency of infections.[113,130] However, since inhibition of the immune system after physical stress is a general phenomenon, which is highly preserved in animals of several species, it is obvious to ask if there are any benefits in poststress immunosuppression. An educated guess or hypothesis could be that if physical stress is associated with tissue damage, the possibility exists that new antigens may be presented to the immune system. The benefit may therefore be that by developing poststress immunosuppression, autoimmune reactions are avoided.[41]

References

1. McCarthy DA, Dale MM. The leucocytosis of exercise. A review and model. Sports Med 1988; 6(6):333-363.
2. Brahmi Z, Thomas JE, Park M et al. The effect of acute exercise on natural killer-cell activity of trained and sedentary human subjects. J Clin Immunol 1985; 5(5):321-328.
3. Fiatarone MA, Morley JE, Bloom ET et al. Endogenous opioids and the exercise-induced augmentation of natural killer cell activity. J Lab Clin Med 1988; 112(5):544-552.
4. Field CJ, Gougeon R, Marliss EB. Circulating mononuclear cell numbers and function during intense exercise and recovery. J Appl Physiol 1991; 71(3):1089-97.
5. Fry RW, Morton AR, Crawford GP et al. Cell numbers and in vitro responses of leukocytes and lymphocyte subpopulations following maximal exercise and interval training sessions of different intensities. Eur J Appl Physiol 1992; 64(3):218-27.
6. Fry RW, Morton AR, Keast D. Acute intensive interval training and T-lymphocyte function. Med Sci Sports Exerc 1992; 24(3):339-45.
7. Gabriel H, Kullmer T, Schwarz L et al. Circulating leukocyte subpopulations in sedentary subjects following graded maximal exercise with hypoxia. Eur J Appl Physiol 1993; 67(4):348-53.
8. Gabriel H, Urhausen A, Kindermann W. Circulating leukocyte and lymphocyte subpopulations before and after intensive endurance exercise to exhaustion. Eur J Appl Physiol 1991; 63(6):449-57.
9. Gabriel H, Urhausen A, Kindermann W. Mobilization of circulating leukocyte and lymphocyte subpopulations during and after short, anaerobic exercise. Eur J Appl Physiol 1992; 65(2):164-70.

10. Hoffman-Goetz L, Simpson JR, Cipp N et al. Lymphocyte subset responses to repeated submaximal exercise in men. J Appl Physiol 1990; 68(3):1069-1074.
11. Kappel M, Tvede N, Galbo H et al. Evidence that the effect of physical exercise on NK cell activity is mediated by epinephrine. J Appl Physiol 1991; 70(6):2530-4.
12. Tvede N, Kappel M, Halkjaer Kristensen J et al. The effect of light, moderate and severe bicycle exercise on lymphocyte subsets, natural and lymphokine activated killer cells, lymphocyte proliferative response and interleukin-2 production. Int J Sports Med 1993; 14(5):275-82.
13. Cannon JG, Fielding RA, Fiatarone MA et al. Increased interleukin 1 beta in human skeletal muscle after exercise. Am J Physiol 1989; 257(2 Pt 2):R451-5.
14. Tvede N, Kappel M, Klarlund K et al. Evidence that the effect of bicycle exercise on blood mononuclear cell proliferative responses and subsets is mediated by epinephrine. Int J Sports Med 1994; 15(2):100-104.
15. Tvede N, Pedersen BK, Hansen FR et al. Effect of physical exercise on blood mononuclear cell subpopulations and in vitro proliferative responses. Scand J Immunol 1989; 29(3):383-389.
16. Lewicki R, Tchorzewski H, Majewska E et al. Effect of Maximal Physical Exercise on T-Lymphocyte Subpopulations and on Interleukin 1 (IL-1) and Interleukin 2 (IL-2) Production in Vitro. Int J Sports Med 1988; 9:114-117.
17. Nieman DC, Henson DA, Johnson R et al. Effects of brief, heavy exertion on circulating lymphocyte subpopulations and proliferative response. Med Sci Sports Exerc 1992; 24(12):1339-1345.
18. Nehlsen Cannarella SL, Nieman DC, Jessen J et al. The effects of acute moderate exercise on lymphocyte function and serum immunoglobulin levels. Int J Sports Med 1991; 12(4):391-398.
19. Nieman DC, Nehlsen Cannarella SL. The effects of acute and chronic exercise of immunoglobulins. Sports Med 1991; 11(3):183-201.
20. Nieman DC, Miller AR, Henson DA et al. Effects of high- vs. moderate-intensity exercise on natural killer cell activity. Med Sci Sports Exerc 1993; 25(10):1126-1134.
21. Ullum H, Palmø J, Halkjaer Kristensen J et al. The effect of acute exercise on lymphocyte subsets, natural killer cells, proliferative responses and cytokines in HIV-seropositive persons. J Acquir Immune Defic Syndr 1994; 7(11):1122-1133.
22. Tvede N, Heilmann C, Halkjaer Kristensen J et al. Mechanisms of B-lymphocyte suppression induced by acute physical exercise. J Clin Lab Immunol 1989; 30(4):169-173.

23. Pedersen BK, Tvede N, Hansen FR et al. Modulation of natural killer cell activity in peripheral blood by physical exercise. Scand J Immunol 1988; 27(6):673-678.
24. Pedersen BK, Tvede N, Klarlund K et al. Indomethacin in vitro and in vivo abolishes postexercise suppression of natural killer cell activity in peripheral blood. Int J Sports Med 1990; 11(2):127-131.
25. Shinkai S, Shore S, Shek PN et al. Acute exercise and immune function. Relationship between lymphocyte activity and changes in subset counts. Int J Sports Med 1992; 13(6):452-61.
26. Edwards AJ, Bacon TH, Elms CA et al. Changes in the populations of lymphoid cells in human peripheral blood following physical exercise. Clin Exp Immunol 1984; 58:420-427.
27. Deuster PA, Curiale AM, Cowan ML et al. Exercise-induced changes in populations of peripheral blood mononuclear cells. Med Sci Sports Exerc 1988; 20:276-280.
28. O'Shea J, Ortaldo JR. The biology of natural killer cells: insights into the molecular basis of function. In: Lewis CE, McGee JO, eds. The Natural Killer Cell. Oxford: Oxford University Press, 1992:1-40.
29. Welsh RM, Vargas-Cortes. Natural killer cells in viral infection. In: Lewis CE, McGee JO, eds. The Natural Killer Cell. Oxford: Oxford University Press, 1992:108-150.
30. Ortaldo JR, Mantovani A, Hobbs D et al. Effects of several species of human leukocyte interferon on cytotoxic activity of NK cells and monocytes. Int J Cancer 1983; 31(3):285-289.
31. Ortaldo JR, Gerard JP, Hendersson LE et al. Responsiveness of purified natural killer cells to pure interleukin 2 (IL-2). In: Oppenheim JJ, Rabin H, eds. Interleukines, Lymphokines and Cytokines. New York: Academic Press, 1983:63-68.
32. Brunda MJ, Herberman RB, Holden HT. Inhibition of murine natural killer cell activity by prostaglandins. J Immunol 1980; 124(6):2682-2687.
33. Pedersen BK, Thomsen BS, Nielsen H. Inhibition of natural killer cell activity by antigen-antibody complexes. Allergy 1986; 41(8):568-574.
34. Grimm EA, Mazumder A, Zhang HZ et al. Lymphokine-activated killer cell phenomenon. Lysis of natural killer-resistant fresh solid tumor cells by interleukin 2-activated autologous human peripheral blood lymphocytes. J Exp Med 1982; 155(6):1823-1841.
35. Whiteside TL, Herberman RB. The role of natural killer cells in human disease. Clin Immunol Immunopathol 1989; 53(1):1-23.
36. Welsh RM. Regulation of virus infections by natural killer cells. A review. Nat Immun Cell Growth Regul 1986; 5(4):169-199.

37. Klokker M, Kjaer M, Secher NH et al. Natural killer cell response to exercise in humans: effect of hypoxia and epidural anesthesia. J Appl Physiol 1995; 78(2):709-16.
38. Klokker M, Secher NH, Matzen S et al. Natural killer cell activity during head-up tilt-induced central hypovolemia in humans. Aviat Space Environ Med 1993; 64(12):1128-1132.
39. Klokker M, Kharazmi A, Galbo H et al. Influence of in vivo hypobaric hypoxia on function of lymphocytes, neutrocytes, natural killer cells and cytokines. J Appl Physiol 1993; 74(3):1100-1106.
40. Kappel M, Stadeager C, Tvede N et al. Effects of in vivo hyperthermia on natural killer cell activity, in vitro proliferative responses and blood mononuclear cell subpopulations. Clin Exp Immunol 1991; 84(1):175-180.
41. Pedersen BK, Kappel M, Klokker M et al. The immune system during exposure to extreme physiologic conditions. Int J Sports Med 1994; 15:S116-21.
42. Espersen GT, Elbaek A, Ernst E et al. Effect of physical exercise on cytokines and lymphocyte subpopulations in human peripheral blood. APMIS 1990; 98(5):395-400.
43. Gabriel H, Schwarz L, Born P et al. Differential mobilization of leukocyte and lymphocyte subpopulations into the circulation during endurance exercise. Eur J Appl Physiol 1992; 65(6):529-34.
44. Haq A, al Hussein K, Lee J et al. Changes in peripheral blood lymphocyte subsets associated with marathon running. Med Sci Sports Exerc 1993; 25(2):186-90.
45. Nieman DC, Nehlsen Cannarella SL, Donohue KM et al. The effects of acute moderate exercise on leukocyte and lymphocyte subpopulations. Med Sci Sports Exerc 1991; 23(5):578-85.
46. Targan S, Britvan L, Dorey F. Activation of human NKCC by moderate exercise: increased frecuency of NK cells with enhanced capability of effector-target lytic interactions. Clin Exp Immunol 1981; 45:352-360.
47. Blank SE, Johansson JO, Origines MM et al. Modulation of NK cell activity by moderate intensity endurance training and chronic ethanol consumption. J Appl Physiol 1992; 72(1):8-14.
48. Bouix O, ElMezouini M, Orsetti A. Effects of naloxone opiate blockade on the immunomodulation induced by exercise in rats. Int J Sports Med 1995; 16(1):29-33.
49. Landmann R. Beta-adrenergic receptors in human leukocyte subpopulations. Eur J Clin Invest 1992; 22(Suppl 1):30-6.
50. Nieman DC, Henson DA, Herring J et al. Natural killer cell cytotoxic activity in weight trainers and sedentary controls. J Strength Cond Res 1994; 8(4):251-4.

51. Peters C, Lotzerich H, Niemeier B et al. Influence of a moderate exercise training on natural killer cytotoxicity and personality traits in cancer patients. Anticancer Res 1994; 14(3A):1033-6.
52. Shephard RJ, Rhind S, Shek PN. Exercise and training: influences on cytotoxicity, interleukin-1, interleukin-2 and receptor structures. Int J Sports Med 1994; 15:S154-66.
53. Palm¢ J, Asp S, Daugaard JR et al. Effect of eccentric exercise on natural killer cell activity. J Appl Physiol 1995; 78(4):1442-1446.
54. Nielsen HB, Secher N, Perdersen BK. Lymphocytes and NK cell activity during repeated bouts of maximal exercise. Am J Physiol 1996; 271:R222-R227.
55. Nielsen HB, Secher NH, Kappel M et al. Lymphocyte, NK and LAK cell responses to maximal exercise. Int J Sports Med 1996; 17:60-65.
56. Rhind SG, Shek PN, Shinkai S et al. Differential expression of interleukin-2 receptor alpha and beta chains in relation to natural killer cell subsets and aerobic fitness. Int J Sports Med 1994; 15(6):911-8.
57. Nieman DC, Henson DA, Sampson CS et al. The acute immune response to exhaustive resistance exercise. Int J Sports Med 1995; 16(5):322-328.
58. Pedersen BK, Ullum H. NK cell response to physical activity: possible mechanisms of action. Med Sci Sports Exerc 1994; 26(2):140-6.
59. Ullum H, Gotzsche PC, Victor J et al. Defective natural immunity: an early manifestation of human immunodeficiency virus infection. J Exp Med 1995; 182(3):789-799.
60. Mackinnon LT. Exercise and Natural Killer Cells What is the Relationship? Sports Med 1989; 7:141-149.
61. Droller MJ, Perlmann P, Schneider MU. Enhancement of natural and antibody-dependent lymphocyte cytotoxicity by drugs which inhibit prostaglandin production by tumor target cells. Cell Immunol 1978; 39(1):154-164.
62. Hall TJ, Brostoff J. Inhibition of human natural killer cell activity by prostaglandin D2. Immunol Lett 1983; 7(3):141-144.
63. Pedersen BK, Oxholm P, Klarlund K. Characterization of the in vivo and in vitro effects of indomethacin on human natural killer cell activity. Allergy 1986; 41(7):532-536.
64. Pedersen BK, Kharazmi A, Svenson M. Downregulation of natural killer cell activity by autologous polymorphonuclear leucocytes. Role of indomethacin. Allergy 1988; 43(1):17-23.
65. Nieman DC, Ahle JC, Henson DA et al. Indomethacin does not alter the natural killer cell response to 2.5 hours of running. J Appl Physiol 1996; 79(3):748-755.

66. Nehlsen Cannarella SL, Nieman DC, Balk Lamberton AJ et al. The effects of moderate exercise training on immune response. Med Sci Sports Exerc 1991; 23(1):64-70.
67. Smith J, Chi D, Salazar S et al. Effect of moderate exercise on proliferative responses of peripheral blood mononuclear cells. J Sports Med Phys Fit 1993; 33(2):152-158.
68. Verde T, Thomas S, Shephard RJ. Potential markers of heavy training in highly trained distance runners. Br J Sports Med 1992; 26(3):167-75.
69. Rohde T, MacLean DA, Hartkopp A et al. The relationship between plasma glutamine level and cellular immune responses in relation to triatlon race. Eur J Appl Physiol 1996; (in press).
70. Espersen ET, Stamp I, Jensen ML et al. Lymphocyte redistribution in connection with physical activity in the rat. Acta Physiol Scand 1995; 155:313-321.
71. Janeway CA, Travers P. The Immune System in Health and Disease. Oxford: Garland Publishing Inc., 1994.
72. Ferry A, Rieu P, Laziri F et al. Immunomodulations of thymocytes and splenocytes in trained rats. J Appl Physiol 1991; 71(3):815-20.
73. Ferry A, Weill B, Amiridis I et al. Splenic immunomodulation with swimming-induced stress in rats. Immunol Lett 1991; 29(3):261-4.
74. Eskola J, Ruuskanen O, Soppi E et al. Effect of sport stress on lymphocyte transformation and antibody formation. Clin Exp Immunol 1978; 32(2):339-345.
75. Espersen GT, Toft E, Ernst E et al. Changes of polymorphonuclear granulocyte migration and lymphocyte proliferative responses in elite runners undergoing intense exercise. Scand J Med Sci Sports 1991; 1:158-62.
76. Fry RW, Morton AR, Garcia Webb P et al. Biological responses to overload training in endurance sports. Eur J Appl Physiol 1992; 64(4):335-44.
77. MacNeil B, Hoffman-Goetz L, Kendall A et al. Lymphocyte proliferation responses after exercise in men: fitness, intensity and duration effects. J Appl Physiol 1991; 70(1):179-85.
78. Rohde T, Ullum H, Palmo J et al. Effects of glutamine on the immune system- influence of muscular exercise and HIV infection. J Appl Physiol 1995; 79(1):146-150.
79. Ortega E, Collazos ME, Barriga C et al. Effect of physical activity stress on the phagocytic process of peritoneal macrophages from old guinea pigs. Mech Ageing Dev 1992; 65(2-3):157-65.
80. Gillis S, Ferm MM, Ou W et al. T cell growth factor: parameters of production and a quantitative microassay for activity. J Immunol 1978; 120(6):2027-2032.

81. Cantrell DA, Smith KA. Transient expression of interleukin 2 receptors. Consequences for T cell growth. J Exp Med 1983; 158(6):1895-1911.
82. Fujii M, Sugamura K, Sano K et al. High-affinity receptor-mediated internalization and degradation of interleukin 2 in human T cells. J Exp Med 1986; 163(3):550-562.
83. Mackinnon LT, Hooper S. Mucosal (secretory) immune system responses to exercise of varying intensity and during overtraining. Int J Sports Med 1994; 15:S179-83.
84. Bierman HR, Kelly KH, Cordes FL et al. The influence of respiratory movements upon the circulating leukocytes. Blood 1952; 7:533-544.
85. Dufaux B, Order U. Complement activation after prolonged exercise. Clin Chim Acta 1989; 179:45-49.
86. Liew FY, Russell SM, Appleyard G et al. Cross-protection in mice infected with influenza A virus by the respiratory route is correlated with local IgA antibody rather than serum antibody or cytotoxic T cell reactivity. Eur J Immunol 1984; 14(4):350-356.
87. Tomasi TB, Trudeau FB, Czerwinski D et al. Immune parameters in athletes before and after strenuous exercise. J Clin Immunol 1982; 2(3):173-178.
88. Mackinnon LT, Chick TW, van As A et al. The effect of exercise on secretory and natural immunity. Adv Exp Med Biol 1987; 216A:869-876.
89. Tharp GD, Barnes MW. Reduction of saliva immunoglobulin levels by swim training. Eur J Appl Physiol 1990; 60(1):61-64.
90. Muns G, Liesen H, Riedel H et al. Influence of long-distance running on IgA in nasal secretion and saliva. Dtsch Z Sportmed 1989; 40:94-99.
91. McDowell SL, Hughes RA, Hughes RJ et al. The effect of exhaustive exercise on salivary immunoglobulin A. J Sports Med Phys Fit 1992; 32(4):412-5.
92. Housh TJ, Johnson GO, Housh DJ et al. The effect of exercise at various temperatures on salivary levels of immunoglobulin A. Int J Sports Med 1991; 12(5):498-500.
93. McDowell SL, Chaloa K, Housh TJ et al. The effect of exercise intensity and duration on salivary immunoglobulin A. Eur J Appl Physiol 1991; 63(2):108-111.
94. Ullum H, Haahr PM, Diamant M et al. Bicycle exercise enhances plasma IL-6 but does not change IL-1α, IL-1β, IL-6, or TNF-α pre-mRNA in BMNC. J Appl Physiol 1994; 77(1):93-7.
95. Cannon JG, Meydani SN, Fielding RA et al. Acute phase response in exercise. II. Associations between vitamin E, cytokines and muscle proteolysis. Am J Physiol 1991; 260(6 Pt 2):R1235-40.

96. Cannon JG, Evans WJ, Hughes VA et al. Physiological mechanisms contributing to increased interleukin-1 secretion. J Appl Physiol 1986; 61(5):1869-1874.
97. Evans WJ, Meredith CN, Cannon JG et al. Metabolic changes following eccentric exercise in trained and untrained men. J Appl Physiol 1986; 61(5):1864-1868.
98. Northoff H, Berg A. Immunologic mediators as parameters of the reaction to strenuous exercise. Int J Sports Med. 1991; 12(Suppl 1):S9-15.
99. Tilz GP, Domej W, Diez Ruiz A et al. Increased immune activation during and after physical exercise. Immunobiol 1993; 188:194-202.
100. Smith JA, Telford RD, Baker MS et al. Cytokine immunoreactivity in plasma does not change after moderate endurance exercise. J Appl Physiol 1992; 73(4):1396-401.
101. Gabriel H, Schmitt B, Urhausen A et al. Increased CD45RA$^+$. Med Sci Sports Exerc 1993; 25(12):1352-7.
102. Dufaux B, Muller R, Hollmann W. Assessment of circulating immune complexes by a solid-phase C1q-binding assay during the first hours and days after prolonged exercise. Clin Chim Acta 1985; 145:313-317.
103. Thomsen BS, Rodgaard A, Tvede N et al. Levels of complement receptor type one (CR1, CD35) on erythrocytes, circulating immune complexes and complement C3 split products C3d and C3c are not changed by short-term physical exercise or training. Int J Sports Med 1992; 13(2):172-5.
104. Simpson IJ, Myles MJ, Smith GW. Immune complexes in normal subjects. J Clin Lab Immunol 1983; 11(3):119-122.
105. Camus G, Duchateau J, Deby Dupont G et al. Anaphylatoxin C5a production during short-term submaximal dynamic exercise in man. Int J Sports Med 1994; 15(1):32-5.
106. Camus G, Pincemail J, Ledent M et al. Plasma levels of polymorphonuclear elastase and myeloperoxidase after uphill walking and downhill running at similar energy cost. Int J Sports Med 1992; 13(6):443-6.
107. Bruunsgaard H, Hartkopp A, Halkjaer Kristensen J, Pedersen BK. Decreased in vivo cell-mediated immunity, but normal vaccination response following intense, longterm exercise. Med Sci Sports Exerc 1996; (in press).
108. Smith JA. Neutrophils, host defense and inflammation: a double-edged sword. J Leukoc Biol 1994; 56(6):672-686.
109. Smith JA, Telford RD, Mason IB et al. Exercise, Training and Neutrophil Microbicidal Activity. Int J Sports Med 1990; 11:179-187.

110. Weidemann MJ, Smith JA, Gray AB et al. Exercise and the immune system. Today's Life Sci 1992; 24-33.
111. Kurokawa Y, Shinkai S, Torii J et al. Exercise-induced changes in the expression of surface adhesion molecules on circulating granulocytes and lymphocytes subpopulations. Eur J Appl Physiol 1995; 71(2-3):245-252.
110. Smith JA, Gray AB, Pyne DB et al. Submaximal exercise causes both priming and activation of neutrophils. Am J Physiol 1996; (in press).
113. Nieman DC. Exercise, upper respiratory tract infection and the immune system. Med Sci Sports Exerc 1994; 26(2):128-39.
114. Ortega E, Collazos ME, Maynar M et al. Stimulation of the phagocytic function of neutrophils in sedentary men after acute moderate exercise. Eur J Appl Physiol 1993; 66(1):60-4.
115. Smith JA, McKenzie SJ, Telford RD et al. Why does moderate exercise enhance, but intense training depress, immunity? In: Husband, ed. Behavior and Immunity. 1992:155-68.
116. Brines R, Hoffman-Goetz L, Pedersen BK. Can you exercise to make your immune system fitter? Immunol Today 1996; 17(6):252-254.
117. Hack V, Strobel G, Rau JP et al. The effect of maximal exercise on the activity of neutrophil granulocytes in highly trained athletes in a moderate training period. Eur J Appl Physiol 1992; 65(6):520-4.
118. Hack V, Strobel G, Weiss M et al. PMN cell counts and phagocytic activity of highly trained athletes depend on training period. J Appl Physiol 1994; 77(4):1731-5.
119. Lewicki R, Tchorzewski H, Denys A et al. Effect of physical exercise on some parameters of immunity in conditioned sportsmen. Int J Sports Med 1987; 8(5):309-314.
120. Buschmann H, Baumann M. Alterations of cellular immune response during intensive training of event horses. Zentralbl Veterinarmed B 1991; 38(2):90-94.
121. Dufaux B, Order U. Plasma elastase-alpha 1-antitrypsin, neopterin, tumor necrosis factor and soluble interleukin-2 receptor after prolonged exercise. Int J Sports Med 1989; 10:434-438.
122. Busse WW, Anderson CL, Hanson PG et al. The effect of exercise on the granulocyte response to isoproterenol in the trained athlete and unconditioned individual. J Allergy Clin Immunol 1980; 65(5):358-364.
123. Hansen JB, Wilsgard L, Osterud B. Biphasic changes in leukocytes induced by strenuous exercise. Eur J Appl Physiol 1991; 62(3):157-61.
124. Kokot K, Schaefer RM, Teschner M et al. Activation of leukocytes during prolonged physical exercise. Adv Exp Med Biol 1988; 240:57-63.

125. Peters AM, Allsop P, Stuttle AW et al. Granulocyte margination in the human lung and its response to strenuous exercise. Clin Sci 1992; 82(2):237-44.
126. Pabst R. The spleen in lymphocyte migration. Immunol Today 1988; 9(2):43-45.
127. Katafuchi T, Ichijo T, Take S et al. Hypothalamic modulation of splenic natural killer cell activity in rats. J Physiol Lond 1993; 471:209-221.
128. Steel CM, French EB, Aitchison WR. Studies on adrenaline-induced leucocytosis in normal man. I. The role of the spleen and of the thoracic duct. Br J Haematol 1971; 21(4):413-421.
129. Iversen PO, Arvesen BL, Benestad HB. No mandatory role for the spleen in the exercise-induced leukocytosis in man. Clin Sci Colch 1994; 86(5):505-10.
130. Friman G, Ilback NG. Exercise and infection—interaction, risks and benefits. Scand J Med Sci Sports 1992; 2:177-89.

CHAPTER 3

Possible Roles of Stress Hormones in Exercise-Induced Immunomodulation

Bente Klarlund Pedersen, Mogens Kappel and Mads Klokker

The migration and recirculation of lymphocytes permit cells of differing specificity, function and antigen experience to be continuously redeployed throughout the body and regrouped in different tissues.[1] A rather stereotypical set of neuroendocrine pathways are critically involved.[2] The major components of these pathways are the activation of nerves of the autonomic nervous system and the activation of nerves in the paraventricular nucleus. Hormones released from endocrine tissues bind to specific receptors either on a cell membrane or within the cytoplasm of a given cell within organs or tissues, and with the cells of the lymphoid system.[3] Thereby, lymphocytes may be recruited from one place to another or the function of the lymphocytes may be modified. The presence of receptors for endocrine hormones[4] and the anatomic contact between the lymphoid and nervous systems[4] reveal the existence of pathways of communication between the immune system, the nervous system and the endocrine system.[3]

Several everyday life activities, including physical exercise, exemplify these regulatory influences. Exercise is known to produce changes in the immune, nervous and endocrine systems[5] and exercise-induced immunomodulation thus represents a subset of neuroendocrinoimmunology.

There are several lines of evidence suggesting that various forms of physical stressors such as trauma, surgery and myocardial infarction, in general, induce the same kind of alterations in the immune system.[6] Exercise is a quantifiable and reproducible experimental stressor and it has been suggested that exercise is a prototype or a model of stress.[7]

Muscular exercise increases the concentrations of adrenaline, noradrenaline, growth hormone, β-endorphins and cortisol, whereas the concentration of insulin slightly decreases.[5,8,9] Studies where these hormones were infused, hormone receptors were blocked by drugs or the hormone production was inhibited by epidural blockade in relation to physical stress, contribute to our understanding of the mechanisms of action. Based on these studies, a model on the possible roles of stress hormones in exercise-induced immune changes can be proposed.

CATECHOLAMINES

During exercise adrenaline is released from the adrenal medulla and noradrenaline is released from the sympathetic nerve terminals. Arterial plasma concentrations of adrenaline and noradrenaline increase almost linearly with duration of dynamic exercise and exponentially with intensity, when it is expressed relative to the individual's maximal oxygen uptake.[8]

The expression of β-adrenoceptors on T, B and natural killer (NK) cells, macrophages and neutrophils in numerous species provides the molecular basis for these cells to be targets for catecholamine signaling.[4] Beta-receptors on lymphocytes are linked intracellularly to the adenyl cyclase system for generation of c adenosinemonophosphate (AMP) as a second messenger,[10] and the β-adrenoceptor density appears to change in conjunction with lymphocyte activation and differentiation.[11]

It was previously reported that proliferation, antibody production and cytotoxic activity could be reduced by β-adrenergic stimulation and in some cases enhanced by α-adrenergic stimulation.[12-18] From such studies, elevation of intracellular cAMP was viewed as a way to limit lymphocyte proliferation and effector function, thereby suppressing the immune response. However, researchers from several laboratories have been unable to replicate the findings of reduced proliferative responses with doses of catecholamines other than pharmacological.[19,20]

The in vitro effect of adrenaline on NK cell activity has been examined by Katz et al,[18] who demonstrated that human NK cell activity was inhibited by the addition of cAMP inducers directly to target and effector cells in a ^{51}Cr-release assay. More complex effects were reported by Hellstrand et al.[21] They found that pretreatment of lymphocytes with low concentrations of adrenaline (10^{-7} to 10^{-9} M), followed by removal of the drug, increased NK cell activity. Whereas direct addition of adrenaline (10^{-6} M) to the lymphocyte-target cell mixture inhibited the NK cell activity.

In the study by Kappel et al,[22] adrenaline was present during preincubation of mononuclear cells as well as in the NK cell assay. The adrenaline concentration (3.8×10^{-9} M) in vitro was comparable to adrenaline concentrations obtained in the plasma during exercise. We were unable to demonstrate any in vitro effects of adrenaline on NK cells isolated before, during or after adrenaline infusion. Therefore, these results indicate that adrenaline may act primarily by redistributing blood mononuclear cell (BMNC) subsets, rather than directly influencing the activity of the individual NK cells.

In theory, the numbers of adrenergic receptors on the individual lymphocyte subpopulations may determine to which degree the cells are mobilized in response to catecholamines. In accordance with this hypothesis, it has been shown that different subpopulations of BMNC have different numbers of adrenergic receptors.[3,23-25]

NK cells contain the highest number of adrenergic receptors with $CD4^+$ lymphocytes having the lowest number. B lymphocytes and $CD8^+$ lymphocytes are intermediate between NK cells and $CD4^+$ lymphocytes (Fig. 3.1).[3] Dynamic exercise upregulates the β-adrenergic receptor density but only on NK cells (Fig. 3.1).[23] Interestingly, NK cells are more sensitive to exercise and other

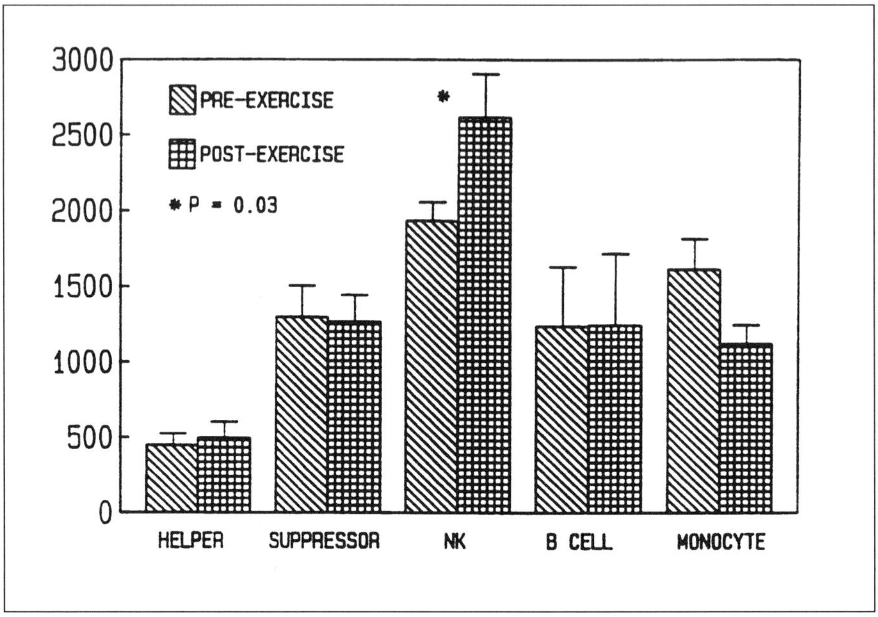

Fig. 3.1. Bar graph showing β-adrenergic density (sites per cell) in lymphocyte subsets of healthy subjects before and after exercise. Values are given as means + SEM of nine individuals. NK, natural killer cells. Reprinted with permission from Maisel AS et al, Circulation 1990; 82:2003-2010.

stressors than any other subpopulation. $CD4^+$ cells are less sensitive and $CD8^+$ cells and B cells are intermediate.[7] Thus, a correlation exists between numbers of adrenergic receptors on lymphocyte subpopulations and their sensitivity to exercise.

In humans, a single adrenaline injection induced transient increases in the number of circulating blood lymphocytes and monocytes and decreased the response to T cell mitogens.[26] Selective intravenous administration of adrenaline to obtain plasma concentrations comparable to those obtained during concentric cycling for 1 hour at 75% of VO_2max, mimicked the exercise-induced effect on blood mononuclear cell subsets, NK cell activity (Fig. 3.2), lymphokine activated killer (LAK) cell activity and the lymphocyte proliferative response (Fig. 3.3).[22,27,28] However, adrenaline infusion caused a significantly smaller increase in neutrophil concentrations than that observed following exercise.[22,27] In addition, we have shown that adrenaline infusion had no effect on the production of interleukin (IL)-1 or tumor necrosis factor-α from BMNC, neither unstimulated nor stimulated with lipopolysaccharide.

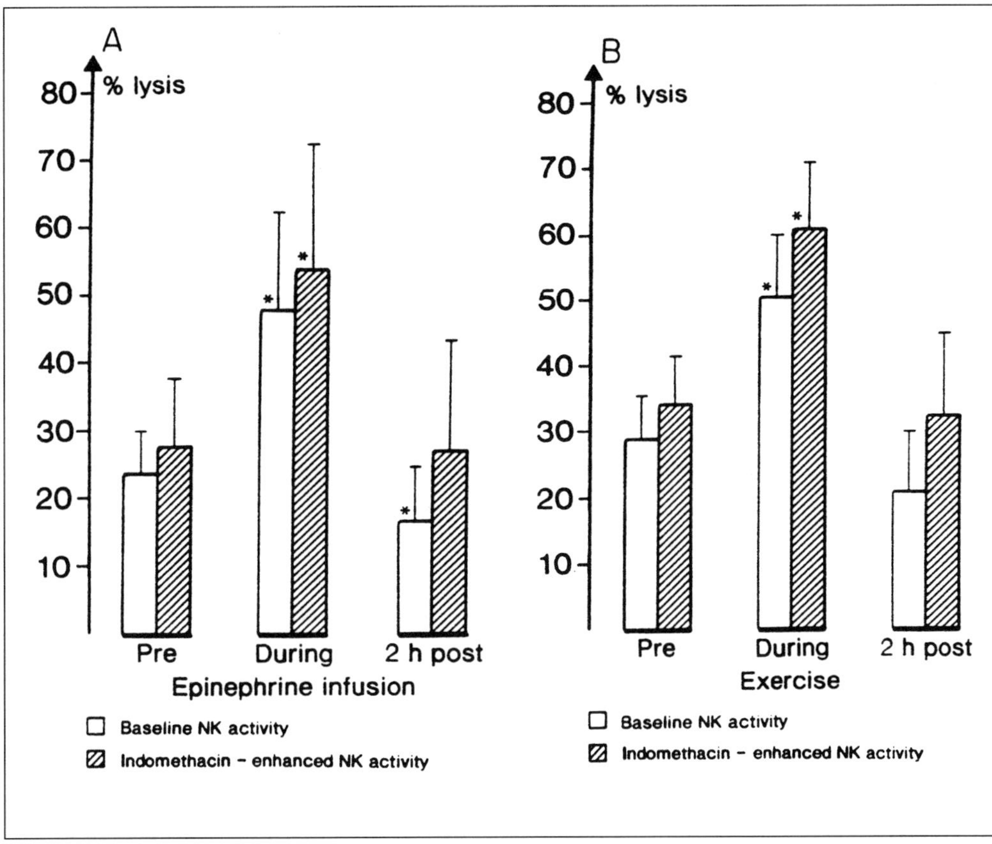

*Fig. 3.2. Natural killer (NK) cell activity against K562 target cells before, during and 2 hours after 60 minutes of intravenous epinephrine infusion (A) and bicycle exercise 75% of VO_2max (B). Blood mononuclear cells were tested in the absence and presence of indomethacin (1 µg/ml). * denotes significant difference from prevalues. Reprinted with permission from Kappel M et al, J Appl Physiol 1991; 70(6):2530-4.*

Ahlborg et al[29] showed that after administration of propranolol, exercise resulted in practically no increase in lymphocyte concentration. Beta 1+2-receptor blockade inhibited head-up tilt-induced lymphocytosis more than β1-blockade (Klokker et al, manuscript submitted for publication). The lymphocytosis during head-up tilt is primarily due to increase in the NK cell subpopulation. The inhibition of head-up tilt-induced lymphocytosis by β1+2 receptor blockade is in accordance with the finding that primarily β2-receptors are expressed on lymphocytes.[30] Beta-receptor blockade did not abolish the head-up tilt-induced neutrocytosis, which is in agreement with previous findings showing that adrenaline infusion caused a smaller increase in neutrophil concentration than the exercise-induced increase.[22,27]

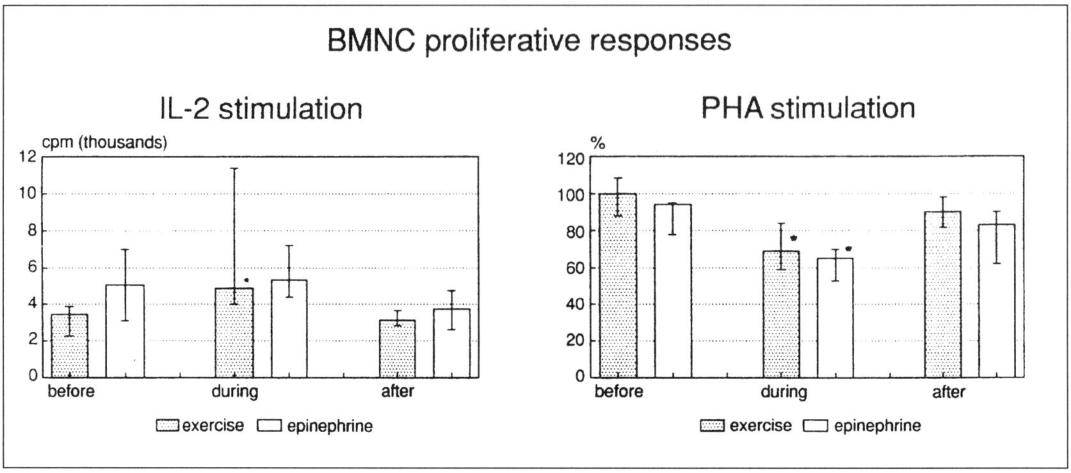

*Fig. 3.3. The effect of 75% of VO_2max bicycle exercise, 1 hour, and epinephrine infusion on blood mononuclear cell (BMNC) proliferative responses. BMNC were incubated with either interleukin (IL)-2 or phytohemagglutinin A (PHA). Medians and quartiles are shown. * denotes significant difference from prevalues. Reprinted with permission from Tvede N et al, Int J Sports Med 1994; 15(2):100-104.*

The effect of noradrenaline on the recruitment of lymphocytes to the blood resembles that of adrenaline, but noradrenaline is far less potent (Kappel et al, manuscript submitted for publication).

The study of the effect of muscular activity on the immune system of subjects with either blockage of afferent or efferent nerve impulses, contributes to our understanding of the links between the nervous, endocrine and immune systems. High cervical cord lesioned individuals (quadriplegia) have an impaired sympathetic nervous system and thereby a reduced catecholamine response to exercise, compared both to normal healthy subjects and to lower thoracic level cord lesioned individuals (paraplegia).[31]

In line with the hypothesis that sympathoadrenergic activity is important especially for the recruitment of NK cells to the blood during exercise, we have recently shown that in relation to electrically stimulated muscular exercise, individuals with quadriplegia have an impaired ability to mobilize NK cells to the blood compared to individuals with paraplegia (Klokker et al, manuscript submitted for publication).

There are several pieces of evidence showing that adrenaline is responsible for the recruitment of NK cells to the blood during physical exercise and other physical stress forms. The experimental basis includes the findings that: (1) adrenaline infusion mimicked the exercise-induced effect especially on NK and LAK cells; (2) the β-adrenergic receptors are upregulated on NK cells during exercise; (3) β-receptor blockade abolished lymphocytosis during exercise and the increase in NK cell number during head-up tilt; (4) spinal cord impaired individuals with impaired sympathoadrenergic activity have an impaired ability to mobilize NK cells to the blood; and (5) β2-receptor-agonists induce selective detachment of NK cells from endothelial cells. The last results strongly support the hypothesis that epinephrine mediates recruitment of NK cells from the marginating pool in blood vessels during stress.

GROWTH HORMONE

Growth hormone is released from the anterior pituitary in a pulsatile manner, and irregular time courses for changes in plasma growth hormone have therefore been found. Plasma levels of pituitary hormones increase in response to exercise both with duration and intensity; however, the growth hormone response is more related to the peak exercise intensity rather than to duration of exercise or total work output.[32,33]

In several species, growth hormone deficiency is associated with small lymphoid organs that have abnormal morphology, and substitution with growth hormone has reconstituted the lymphoid organs, suggesting that growth hormone is important for normal development of the immune system.[4] In agreement with this, there are studies showing that growth hormone reconstitution may modulate the immune system of growth hormone deficient patients.[4] Thus, the NK cell activity has been shown to be depressed in growth hormone deficient individuals[34-37] but longterm (more than 6 weeks) growth hormone administration restored the NK cell activity.[38,39] However, shortterm substitution of growth hormone or growth hormone releasing factor restored the NK cell function in some[35,40] but not all studies.[36,37] Long term growth hormone substitution administered to children did not alter the number[41] or function of granulocytes.[36]

Addressing the question of a possible role of growth hormone in mediating acute exercise induced immune changes, Kappel et al[42] administered an in vivo injection of growth hormone in humans to obtain blood concentrations of growth hormone comparable with those observed during exercise. An intravenous bolus injection of growth hormone had no effect on BMNC subsets, NK cell activity, cytokine production or lymphocyte function, but it induced a highly significant neutrocytosis (Fig. 3.5).[42] Therefore, growth hormone does not seem to play a major role in exercise-induced recruitment of lymphocytes to the blood. However, epinephrine and growth hormone in conjunction are probably responsible for the recruitment of neutrophils to the blood during short time physical stress.

BETA-ENDORPHIN

Beta-endorphin is a peptide hormone belonging to the endogenous opioids. It is produced primarily in the pituitary by degradation of the prohormone β-lipotropin, a fragment of pro-opiomelanocortin. When the N-terminal signal peptide has been removed posttranslatory, enzymatic processes in the anterior pituitary cleave pro-opiomelanocortin into β–lipotropin and adrenocorticotropin (ACTH), a joining peptide and an NH_2-terminal peptide. Some of the β-lipotropin is then cleaved into γ-lipotropin and β-endorphin. In the intermediate pituitary almost all β-lipotropin is degraded into these two peptides. For example, with a half life in human plasma of approximately 45 minutes β-endorphin is relatively stable compared to the enkephalins.

At rest the circulating level of β-endorphin is 1-100 $\times 10^{-12}$ M, but several kinds of stress such as fear, physical activity, pregnancy and labor increase the level 3-10 times.[23,42] The plasma concentrations of β-endorphin increase in response to prolonged exercise if the intensity is above 50% of VO_2max and during maximal exercise if this is performed for a minimum of 3 minutes. At low work loads no rise in β-endorphin levels were found despite extremely long exposure time.[43-47]

The explosion of knowledge that followed the first identification of endogenous opioid peptides, makes it difficult to integrate the various and often contrasting data in a single theory. However, without doubt the opioid system influences the immune response. Functional evidence for opioid receptors on human T lymphocytes was first reported by Wybran[45] after which numerous reports have appeared (reviewed by Madden and Felten).[4]

At present, a clear functional role has not yet emerged for the opioid peptides. The reasons for this lack of agreement may be related to the heterogeneity of the opioid peptides and receptors. Furthermore, some effects of opioids are blocked by opioid receptor blockers such as naloxone, whereas other effects are not.[4]

The results on β-endorphin and T cell function are highly variable. However, the studies by van den Berg[48] contribute to the divergent findings regarding T cell proliferation. Based on studies performed in humans, and weighing the experiments, where β-endorphin was continuously present, β-endorphin seems to inhibit T cell proliferation.

Most studies suggest that β-endorphin inhibits antibody-production. This inhibitory effect of β-endorphin can probably be ascribed to interaction with opioid receptors as the N-terminal of the molecule is necessary to induce the inhibition and since this inhibition can be blocked by naloxone.[49]

Both interferon (IFN) and IL-2 stimulate NK cells to increased cytotoxic activity. If incubated with human BMNC or NK-enriched cell populations, β-endorphin is able to enhance the NK activity by 10-15%.[50,51] However, other investigations do not yield such unambiguous results. It has been found that β-endorphin in many cases only stimulates the NK cell activity among some of the donors.[52] Additionally this activity may be inhibited by β-endorphin.[53,54] Even day-to-day variations have been seen with a number of donors.[54]

The NK cell activity shows a circadian rhythm with maximal activity around 6 a.m. and a minimal activity around 6 p.m. Likewise the level of β-endorphin reaches its maximum and minimum in the morning and in the evening, respectively.[55] Hence, this level fluctuates in phase with the cytolytic activity of the NK cells indicating that β-endorphin may have a stimulating effect on the NK cells. In order to draw any conclusions from studies of circadian rhythms it is, however, necessary to determine the 24 hour fluctuations of other known modulators of the NK cell cytolytic activity (e.g., IFN, cortisol or catecholamines). Beta-endorphin enhances the production of IFN by NK cells[56] and by other BMNC[57] and may thereby create a positive feed-back mechanism. In summary, although there are divergent findings, most studies indicate that β-endorphin enhances the NK cell activity, it is not known whether β-endorphin influences the NK cell activity by recruitment of effector cells, by increasing the adhesion (the number of effector cell-target cell conjugates) or by enhancing the lytic step.

It is evident that β-endorphin plays a considerable role in the regulation of the immune system. However, in addition, some cytokines also influence the production and release of β-endorphin from the pituitary. Both IL-1 and IL-2 are able to cross the blood brain barrier under certain conditions.[58,59] They have also been shown to augment corticotropin releasing factor and vasopressin induced β-endorphin production and secretion in the pituitary. An IL-2 receptor has in fact been found in the rat hypothalamus.[59] Moreover, some studies indicate that IL-1 directly influences the anterior pituitary cells and thereby induces production of β-endorphin.[60-62]

In order to explore the possibility that the rise in β-endorphin during exercise was responsible for the exercise-induced increase in NK cell activity, Fiatarone et al[63] administered naloxone in vivo to young women who underwent a maximal cycle ergometer test. In the naloxone experiment, the rise in NK cell activity was no longer significant. However, the exercise-induced increase in cells expressing the CD16 marker (NK cells) was not significantly altered compared with the group receiving placebo.

Employing another physical stress model, it was shown that naloxone in vivo had no effect on head-up tilt induced recruitment of NK cells to the circulation. Beta-endorphin receptor blockade also had no influence on the function of NK cells or any other subpopulations of BMNC (Klokker et al, manuscript submitted for publication). Furthermore, naloxone in vivo had no effect on hyperthermia-induced recruitment of NK cells to the blood (Kappel et al, manuscript submitted for publication).

Afferent nerve impulses can be blocked by epidural analgesia (Fig. 3.4). Thereby the increases in β-endorphins and ACTH are inhibited during exercise. In a study by Klokker et al,[64] the exercise-induced increase in NK cell function, percentage of NK cells and NK cell concentration were significantly enlarged in the experiment where the afferent nerve impulses were inhibited (Fig. 3.6).[64] Thus, it seems that blocking the β-endorphin receptor[63] and blocking the increase in concentration of β-endorphin[64] during exercise exert differential effects on the immune system.

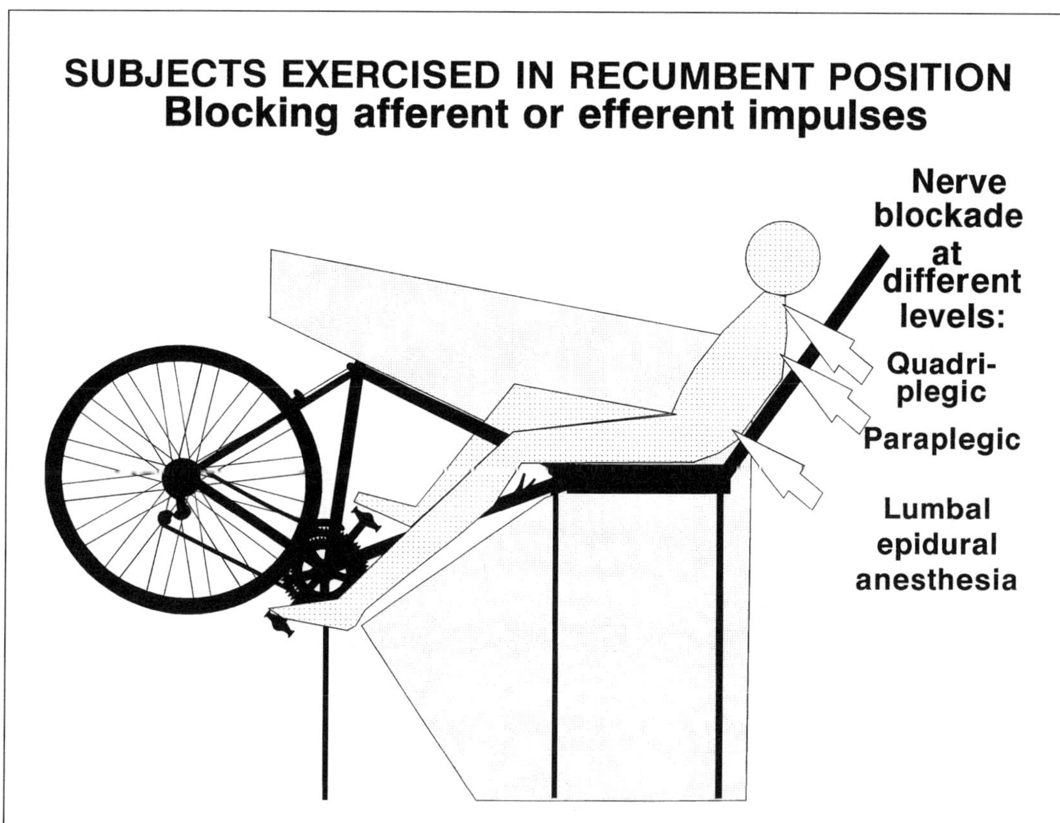

Fig. 3.4. Schematic representation of experimental designs allowing researchers to study the importance of afferent and efferent nerve impulses for exercise-induced immunomodulation. Nerve blockade can be due either to anaesthesiological blockade (blocking afferent nerve impulses) or due to cervical cord lesion at different levels (e.g., as seen in paraplegic and quadriplegic individuals).

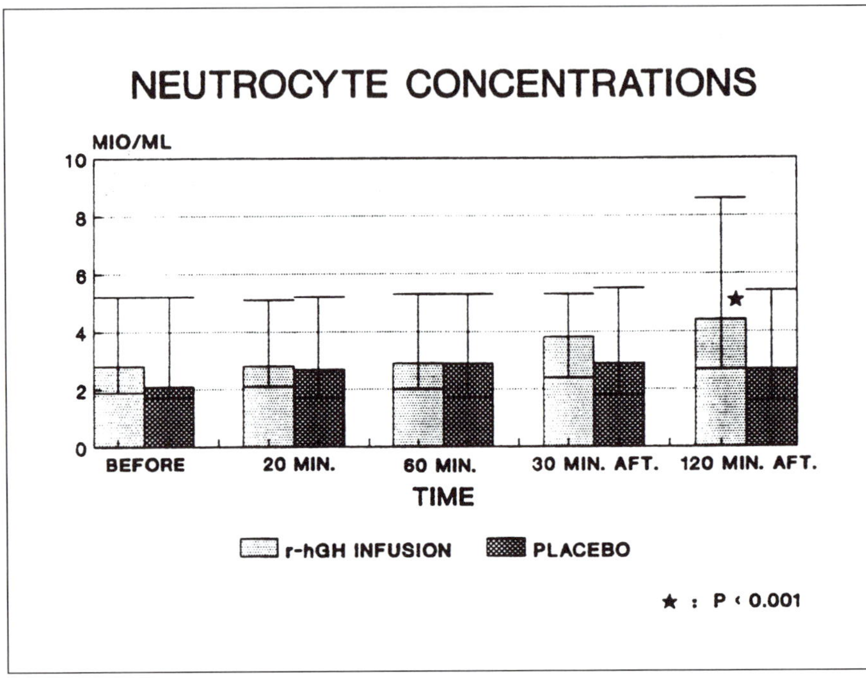

*Fig. 3.5. The effect of an acute bolus recombinant growth hormone (r-GH) infusion for 1 hour on neutrocyte concentrations before, at 20 minutes and 60 minutes, as well as 30 minutes and 120 minutes after r-GH infusion (Medians and extreme values). * denotes significant difference ($p < 0.001$). Reprinted with permission from Kappel M et al, Horm Metab Res 1993; 25(11):579-585.*

Animal experiments showed that chronic intracerebrovascular infusion of β-endorphin augments the NK cell activity in vivo and that this effect was abolished by naloxone.[65] It was concluded that this effect was centrally- and opioid- receptor mediated, since β-endorphin in the same dose administered peripherally did not influence in vivo NK cell cytotoxicity.

It is not easy to determine exactly what role β-endorphin has in exercise-induced immunomodulation. However, the available data indicates that β-endorphin is not responsible for the immediate recruitment of NK cells to the blood during acute exercise, but likely responsible for increased NK cell activity during chronic stress. This is based on the fact that NK cells are recruited to the blood immediately after the onset of exercise and even at exercise of very low intensity. Whereas the concentrations of β-endorphin increase only at high intensity and long duration exercise, which make it unlikely that β-endorphin plays a major immunomodulatory role

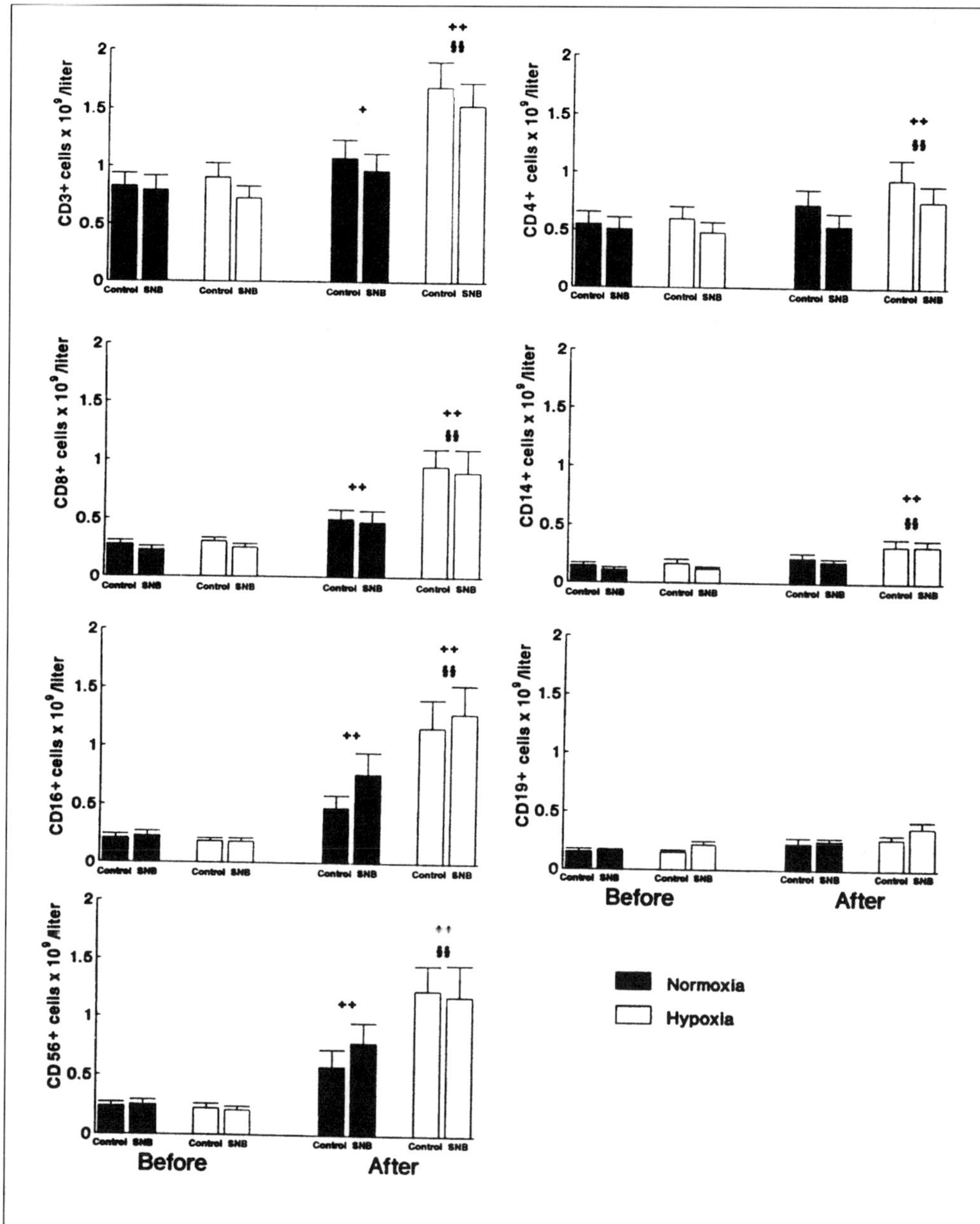

*Fig. 3.6 Blood mononuclear cell (BMNC) subset concentrations at normoxic (solid bars) and hypoxic cycling (open bars), compared with time (before and after exercise) without (control) and with sensory nervous blockade (SNB). Blood samples were collected before and after cycling. Values are given as means and SEM, n = experiments. Tukey's post hoc test based on analysis of variance (ANOVA) disclosing significant estimated interaction effects (Exercise*Hypoxia) + $p < 0.05$ and ++$p < 0.01$ denote significant difference between before and after values at normoxia and hypoxia. §§ $p < 0.01$ denotes significant difference between normoxia and hypoxia. Reprinted with permission from Klokker M et al, J Appl Physiol 1995; 78(2):709-16.*

in the immediate recruitment of NK cells to the blood. Furthermore, Fiatarone et al[63] reported that naloxone blocked the exercise-induced increase in NK cell activity; the differences were, although statistically significant, small, and there was no effect of β-endorphin receptor blockade on the number of cells.

The finding that β-endorphin receptor blockade during head-up tilt and anaesthesiological inhibition of the exercise-induced increase in β-endorphin do not inhibit the recruitment of NK cells to the blood,[64] further supports the idea that β-endorphin does not play a role in the immediate recruitment of NK cells during acute exercise. The hypothesis that β-endorphin is important in maintaining increased NK cell activity during chronic stress is primarily based on animal studies showing that voluntary chronic exercise augments in vivo natural immunity.[65,66] In addition β-endorphin and dynorphin in hypertensive rats[65,67,68] and β-endorphin infusion, but not infusion of dynorphin to rats, increased the NK cell activity.[65]

CORTISOL

The plasma concentrations of cortisol increases only in relation to exercise of long duration.[9] Thus, short term exercise does not increase the cortisol concentration in plasma, and only minor changes in the concentrations of plasma cortisol was described in relation to acute time-limited exercise stress of 1 hour.[9]

The effect on the immune system of corticosteroids in vivo has been described by several authors.[3,69] Corticosteroids exert their effects on the immune system with a time lag of several hours. Glucocorticoids are able to enter the cytoplasm of cells and bind to glucocorticoid receptors.[3] It has been shown that corticosteroids given intravenously to humans cause lymphocytopenia, monocytopenia, eosinopenia and neutrocytosis which reach their maximum 4 hours after administration.

Exogenous glucocorticosteroid administration, especially in supraphysiological doses, induces cell death of immature T and B cells, whereas mature T cells and activated B cells are relatively resistant to cell death.[70] Cox and Ford[71] demonstrated that infusion of prednisolone caused a redistribution of circulating cells from blood to the bone marrow, decreased cellular localization to lymph nodes and impaired lymphocyte crossing of endothelial venules.

Parillo and Fauchi[72] found that 12 mg of the long acting preparation of oral dexamethasone decreased NK cell activity at 24 and 48 hours, with normalization by 96 hours. Onsrud and Thorsby[73] as well as Katz et al[74] showed increased NK cell activity at 4 hours after intravenous hydrocortisone, 300 mg and 400 mg, respectively. We reported that methylprednisolone pulse therapy (1 gram intravenously on 4 consecutive days) in patients with rheumatoid arthritis produced a considerable fall in the NK cell activity during methylprednisolone pulse therapy lasting 3 months. This indicated that suprapharmacological concentrations of methylprednisolone induced irreversible inhibition of the NK cell activity.[75]

In vitro studies have shown that pharmacological concentrations of methylprednisolone and hydrocortisone inhibited NK cell function, partly by an inhibition of the adhesion of effector cells to target cells.[76,77] Glucocortioids also inhibit mitogen- and alloantigen-stimulated T cell proliferation in vitro through cytoplasmic glucocorticoid receptors in T and B lymphocytes and macrophages.[78-80]

Unlike catecholamines, cortisol exerts its effect with a time-lag of several hours and therefore it can be excluded that cortisol plays a role in the acute exercise-induced effects. Furthermore, only exercise of long duration and intensity induce prolonged changes in the immune system. Therefore, we hypothesize that cortisol plays a role in maintaining the neutrocytosis and lymphopenia after prolonged, intense exercise such as a marathon.

CONCLUSION

Based on these studies we propose a model (Fig. 3.7) on the possible roles of stress hormones in mediating exercise-related immune changes: adrenaline and to a lesser degree noradrenaline are responsible for acute exercise effects on lymphocyte subpopulations and NK and LAK cell activities. The increase in catecholamines and growth hormone mediates the acute effects on neutrophils, whereas cortisol exerts its effects within a time lag of at least 2 hours and contributes to maintain the lymphopenia and neutrocytosis only after longterm exercise. The role of β-endorphin is less clear, but we do not believe that β-endorphin plays an important role in the immediate recruitment of NK cells to the blood. β-endorphin increases after longterm exercise and we can not exclude that it is important in chronic stress. Stress hormones do not seem to be

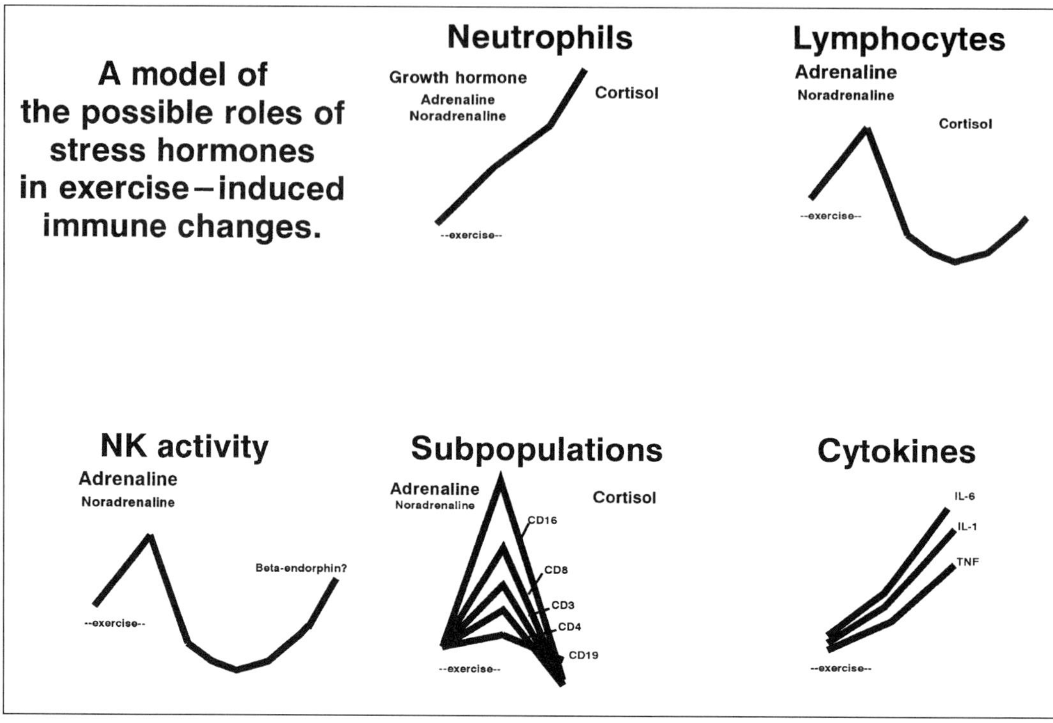

Fig. 3.7. A model of the possible roles of stress hormones in mediating exercise-related immunological changes is proposed. Adrenaline and to a lesser degree noradrenaline are responsible for the acute effects of exercise on lymphocyte count and NK cell activity. Catecholamines and growth hormone in combination are responsible for the effects on neutrocytes. Cortisol contributes to maintain lymphopenia and neutrocytosis only after longterm stress. The role of β-endorphin is less clear, but it has been suggested to play a role in chronic stress.

responsible for the exercise-induced increase in cytokines. This hypothesis is an extension of the hypothesis previously suggested by McCarthy and Dale[81] that the immediate leukocytosis during exercise is attributable to elevated catecholamine levels, whereas the delayed neutrocytosis is due to raised cortisol levels.

References

1. Ottaway CA, Husband AJ. The influence of neuroendocrine pathways on lymphocyte migration. Immunol Today 1994; 15(11):511-517.
2. Johnson EO, Kamilaris TC, Chrousos GP et al. Mechanisms of Stress: A Dynamic Overview of Hormonal and Behavioral Homeostasis. Neurosci Biobehav Rev 1992; 16:115-130.

3. Rabin BS, Moyna MN, Kusnecov A et al. 2, Neuroendocrine effects of immunity. In: Hoffman-Goetz L, ed. Exercise and Immune Function. Boca Raton, New York, London, Tokyo: CRC, 1996:21-38.
4. Madden K, Felten DL. Experimental basis for neural-immune interactions. Physiol Rev 1995; 75:77-77.
5. Kjaer M, Dela F. 1, Endocrine responses to Exercise. In: Hoffman-Goetz L, ed. Exercise and Immune Function. New York: CRC Press, 1996:1-20.
6. Pedersen BK, Kappel M, Klokker M et al. The immune system during exposure to extreme physiologic conditions. Int J Sports Med 1994; 15:S116-21.
7. Hoffman-Goetz L, Pedersen BK. Exercise and the immune system: a model of the stress response? Immunol Today 1994; 15(8):382-7.
8. Kjaer M. Epinephrine and some other hormonal responses to exercise in man: with special reference to physical training. Int J Sports Med 1989; 10(1):2-15.
9. Galbo H. Hormonal and Metabolic Adaption to Exercise. New York: Thieme Verlag, 1983:1-117.
10. Carlson SL, Brooks WH, Roszman TL. Neurotransmitter-lymphocyte interactions: dual receptor modulation of lymphocyte proliferation and cAMP production. J Neuroimmunol 1989; 24(1-2): 155-162.
11. Ackerman KD, Bellinger DL, Felten SY et al.Ontogeny and senescence of noradrenergic innervention of the rodent thymus and spleen. In: Ader R, Felten DL, Cohen N, eds. Psychoneuroimmunology. San Diego: Academic, 1991:71-125.
12. Hadden JW, Hadden EM, Middleton Jr E. Lymphocyte blast transformation. I. Demonstration of adrenergic receptors in human peripheral lymphocytes. Cell Immunol 1970; 1(6):583-595.
13. Johnson DL, Ashmore RC, Gordon MA. Effects of beta-adrenergic agents on the murine lymphocyte response to mitogen stimulation. J Immunopharmacol 1981; 3(2):205-219.
14. Strom TB, Carpenter CB, Garovoy MR et al. The modulating influence of cyclic nucleotides upon lymphocyte-mediated cytotoxicity. J Exp Med 1973; 138(2):381-393.
15. Watson J. The influence of intracellular levels of cyclic nucleotides on cell proliferation and the induction of antibody synthesis. J Exp Med 1975; 141(1):97-111.
16. Melmon KL, Bourne HR, Weinstein Y et al. Hemolytic plaque formation by leukocytes in vitro. Control by vasoactive hormones. J Clin Invest 1974; 53(1):13-21.
17. Goodwin JS, Messner RP, Williams Jr RC. Inhibitors of T-cell mitogenesis: effect of mitogen dose. Cell Immunol 1979; 45(2):303-308.

18. Katz P, Zaytoun AM, Fauci AS. Mechanisms of human cell-mediated cytotoxicity. I. Modulation of natural killer cell activity by cyclic nucleotides. J Immunol 1982; 129(1):287-296.
19. Butler J, Kelly JG, O'Malley K et al. Beta-adrenoceptor adaptation to acute exercise. J Physiol Lond 1983; 344:113-117.
20. Dufaux B, Order U, Geyer H et al. C-reactive protein serum concentrations in well-trained athletes. Int J Sports Med 1984; 5:102-106.
21. Hellstrand K, Hermodsson S, Strannegard O. Evidence for a beta-adrenoceptor-mediated regulation of human natural killer cells. J Immunol 1985; 134(6):4095-4099.
22. Kappel M, Tvede N, Galbo H et al. Evidence that the effect of physical exercise on NK cell activity is mediated by epinephrine. J Appl Physiol 1991; 70(6):2530-4.
23. Maisel AS, Harris C, Rearden CA et al. Beta-adrenergig receptors in lymphocyte subsets after exercise. Alterations in normal individuals and patients with congestive heart failure. Circulation 1990; 82:2003-2010.
24. Khan MM, Sansoni P, Silverman ED et al. Beta-adrenergic receptors on human suppressor, helper and cytolytic lymphocytes. Biochem Pharmacol 1986; 35(7):1137-1142.
25. van Tits LJ, Graafsma SJ. Stress influences $CD4^+$ lymphocyte counts. Immunol Lett 1991; 30(1):141-142.
26. Crary B, Borysenko M, Sutherland DC et al. Decrease in mitogen responsiveness of mononuclear cells from peripheral blood after epinephrine administration in humans. J Immunol 1983; 130(2):694-697.
27. Tvede N, Kappel M, Klarlund K et al. Evidence that the effect of bicycle exercise on blood mononuclear cell proliferative responses and subsets is mediated by epinephrine. Int J Sports Med 1994; 15(2):100-104.
28. Tønnesen E, Christensen NJ, Brinklov MM. Natural killer cell activity during cortisol and adrenaline infusion in healthy volunteers. Eur J Clin Invest 1987; 17(6):497-503.
29. Ahlborg B, Ahlborg G. Exercise leukocytosis with and without beta-adrenergic blockade. Acta Med Scand 1970; 187:241-246.
30. Benschop RJ, Oostveen FG, Heijnen CJ et al. Beta 2-adrenergic stimulation causes detachment of natural killer cells from cultured endothelium. Eur J Immunol 1993; 23(12):3242-3247.
31. Wallin BG, Stjernebjerg T. Sympathetic activity in man after spinal cord injury: Outflow to skin lesion. Brain 1984; 107:183-198.
32. Kjaer M. Regulation of hormonal and metabolic responses during exercise in humans. Exerc Sport Sci Rev 1992; 20:1-11.
33. Vanhelder WP, Radomski MW, Goode RC. Growth hormone responses during intermittent weight lifting exercise in men. Eur J Appl Physiol 1984; 53(1):31-34.

34. Bozzola M, Valtorta A, Moretta A et al. In vitro and in vivo effect of growth hormone on cytotoxic activity. J Pediatr 1990; 117(4):596-599.
35. Crist DM, Peake GT, Mackinnon LT et al. Exogenous growth hormone treatment alters body composition and increases natural killer cell activity in women with impaired endogenous growth hormone secretion. Metabolism 1987; 36(12):1115-1117.
36. Kiess W, Malozowski S, Gelato M et al. Lymphocyte subset distribution and natural killer activity in growth hormone deficiency before and during short-term treatment with growth hormone releasing hormone. Clin Immunol Immunopathol 1988; 48(1):85-94.
37. Kiess W, Doerr H, Eisl E et al. Lymphocyte subsets and natural-killer activity in growth hormone deficiency [letter]. N Engl J Med 1986; 314(5):321-321.
38. Olson GA, Olson RD, Kastin AJ. Endogenous opiates. Peptides 1991; 12(6):1407-1432.
39. Watson J, Epstein R, Cohn M. Cyclic nucleotides as intracellular mediators of the expression of antigen-sensitive cells. Nature 1973; 246(5433):405-409.
40. Matsuura M, Kikkawa Y, Kitagawa T et al. Modulation of immunological abnormalities of growth hormone-deficient children by growth hormone treatment. Acta Paediatr Jpn 1989; 31(1):53-57.
41. Bozzola M, Cisternino M, Valtorta A et al. Effect of biosynthetic methionyl growth hormone (GH) therapy on the immune function in GH-deficient children. Horm Res 1989; 31(4):153-156.
42. Kappel M, Hansen MB, Diamant M et al. Effects of an acute bolus growth hormone infusion on the human immune system. Horm Metab Res 1993; 25(11):579-585.
43. Kraemer WJ, Patton JF, Knuttgen HG et al. Hypothalamic-pituitary-adrenal responses to short-duration high-intensity cycle exercise. J Appl Physiol 1989; 66(1):161-166.
44. Pestell RG, Hurley DM, Vandongen R. Biochemical and hormonal changes during a 1000 km ultramarathon. Clin Exp Pharmacol Physiol 1989; 16(5):353-361.
45. Wybran J, Appelboom T, Famaey JP et al. Suggestive evidence for receptors for morphine and methionine-enkephalin on normal human blood T lymphocytes. J Immunol 1979; 123(3):1068-1070.
46. McMurray RG, Forsythe WA, Mar MH et al. Exercise intensity-related responses of beta-endorphin and catecholamines. Med Sci Sports Exerc 1987; 19(6):570-574.
47. Sforzo GA. Opioids and exercise. An update. Sports Med 1989; 7(2):109-124.
48. van den Bergh P, Rozing J, Nagelkerken L. Identification of two moieties of beta-endorphin with opposing effects on rat T-cell proliferation. Immunology 1993; 79(1):18-23.

49. Morgan EL, McClurg MR, Janda JA. Suppression of human B lymphocyte activation by beta-endorphin. J Neuroimmunol 1990; 28(3):209-217.
50. Mathews PM, Froelich CJ, Sibbitt WL, Jr. et al. Enhancement of natural cytotoxicity by beta-endorphin. J Immunol 1983; 130(4):1658-1662.
51. Kay N, Allen J, Morley JE. Endorphins stimulate normal human peripheral blood lymphocyte natural killer activity. Life Sci 1984; 35(1):53-59.
52. Puente J, Maturana P, Miranda D et al. Enhancement of human natural killer cell activity by opioid peptides: similar response to methionine-enkephalin and beta-endorphin. Brain Behav Immun 1992; 6(1):32-39.
53. Yeager MP, Yu CT, Campbell AS et al. Effect of morphine and beta-endorphin on human Fc receptor-dependent and natural killer cell functions. Clin Immunol Immunopathol 1992; 62(3):336-343.
54. Chiappelli F, Yamashita N, Faisal M et al. Differential effect of beta-endorphin on three human cytotoxic cell populations. Int J Immunopharmacol 1991; 13(2-3):291-297.
55. Mozzanica N, Finzi AF, Foppa S et al. Association between circadian rhythms of endogenous hypothalamic opioid peptides and of natural killer cell activity. Int J Immunopharmacol 1991; 13(2-3):317-321.
56. Mandler RN, Biddison WE, Mandler R et al. beta-Endorphin augments the cytolytic activity and interferon production of natural killer cells. J Immunol 1986; 136(3):934-939.
57. Brown SL, Van Epps DE. Opioid peptides modulate production of interferon gamma by human mononuclear cells. Cell Immunol 1986; 103(1):19-26.
58. Parsadaniantz SM, Lenoir V, Terlain B et al. Lack of effect of interleukins 1 alpha and 1 beta, during in vitro perifusion, on anterior pituitary release of adrenocorticotropic hormone and beta endorphin in the male rat. J Neurosci Res 1993; 34(3):315-323.
59. Lapchak PA, Araujo DM. Interleukin-2 regulates monoamine and opioid peptide release from the hypothalamus. Neuroreport 1993; 4(3):303-306.
60. Fagarasan MO, Arora PK, Axelrod J. Interleukin-1 potentiation of beta-endorphin secretion and the dynamics of interleukin-1 internalization in pituitary cells. Prog. Neuropsychopharmacol. Biol Psychiatry 1991; 15(4):551-560.
61. Lissoni P, Barni S, Rovelli F et al. Neuroendocrine effects of subcutaneous interleukin-2 injection in cancer patients. Tumori 1991; 77(3):212-215.

62. Fagarasan MO, Axelrod J, Catt KJ. Interleukin 1 potentiates agonist-induced secretion of beta-endorphin in anterior pituitary cells. Biochem Biophys Res Commun 1990; 173(3):988-993.
63. Fiatarone MA, Morley JE, Bloom ET et al. Endogenous opioids and the exercise-induced augmentation of natural killer cell activity. J Lab Clin Med 1988; 112(5):544-552.
64. Klokker M, Kjaer M, Secher NH et al. Natural killer cell response to exercise in humans: effect of hypoxia and epidural anesthesia. J Appl Physiol 1995; 78(2):709-16.
65. Jonsdottir IH, Johansson C, Asea A, Hellstrand K, Thoren P, Hoffmann P. Chronic intracerebrovascular administration of Beta-endorphin augments natural killer cell cytotoxicity in rats. Regulatory Peptides 1996; (in press).
66. Jonsdottir IH, Asea A, Hoffmann P et al. Voluntary chronic exercise augments in vivo natural immunity in rats. J Appl Physiol 1996; (in press).
67. Hoffmann P, Terenius L, Thoren P. Cerebrospinal fluid immunoreactive exercise in spontaneously hypertensive rat. Regulatory Peptides 1996; 28:233-239.
68. Persson S, Jonsdottir I, Thoren P et al. Cerebrospinal fluid dynorphin-converting enzyme activity is increased by voluntary exercise in the spontaneously hypertensive rat. Life Sci 1993; 53(8):643-652.
69. Pedersen BK. Modulation of natural killer cell activity in patients with immune-inflammatory diseases. Dan Med Bull 1988; 35(4):315-322.
70. Cohen JJ, Duke RC. Glucocorticoid activation of a calcium-dependent endonuclease in thymocyte nuclei leads to cell death. J Immunol 1984; 132(1):38-42.
71. Cox JH, Ford WL. The migration of lymphocytes across specialized vascular endothelium. IV. Prednisolone acts at several points on the recirculation pathways of lymphocytes. Cell Immunol 1982; 66(2):407-422.
72. Parillo JE, Fauchi AS. Comparison of the effector cells in human spontaneous cellular cytotoxicity: differential sensitivity of effector cells to in vivo and in vitro corticosteroids. Scand J Immunol 1978; 8:99-107.
73. Onsrud M, Thorsby E. Influence of in vivo hydrocortisone on some human blood lymphocyte subpopulations. I. Effect on natural killer cell activity. Scand J Immunol 1981; 13(6):573-579.
74. Katz P, Zaytoun AM, Lee Jr JH. The effects of in vivo hydrocortisone on lymphocyte-mediated cytotoxicity. Arthritis Rheum 1984; 27(1):72-78.

75. Pedersen BK, Beyer JM, Rasmussen A et al. Methylprednisolone pulse therapy induced fall in natural killer cell activity in rheumatoid arthritis. Acta Pathol Microbiol Immunol Scand C 1984; 92(5):319-323.
76. Hoffman T, Hirata F, Bougnoux P et al. Phospholipid methylation and phospholipase A2 activation in cytotoxicity by human natural killer cells. Proc Natl Acad Sci USA 1981; 78(6):3839-3843.
77. Pedersen BK, Beyer JM. Characterization of the in vitro effects of glucocorticosteroids on NK cell activity. Allergy 1986; 41(3):220-224.
78. Cupps TR, Fauci AS. Corticosteroid-mediated immunoregulation in man. Immunol Rev 1982; 65:133-155.
79. Smith KA, Crabtree GR, Kennedy SJ et al. Glucocorticoid receptors and glucocorticoid sensitivity of mitogen stimulated and unstimulated human lymphocytes. Nature 1977; 267(5611):523-526.
80. Werb Z, Foley R, Munck A. Interaction of glucocorticoids with macrophages. Identification of glucocorticoid receptors in monocytes and macrophages. J Exp Med 1978; 147(6):1684-1694.
81. McCarthy DA, Dale MM. The leucocytosis of exercise. A review and model. Sports Med 1988; 6(6):333-363.

CHAPTER 4

Possible Role of Hyperthermia and Hypoxia in Exercise-Induced Immunomodulation

Bente Klarlund Pedersen, Mads Klokker and Mogens Kappel

Two of the physiological changes that occur during dynamic exercise are hyperthermia and oxygen debt. Is it possible that these physiological stimuli are at least partly responsible for exercise-induced immunomodulation?

HYPERTHERMIA

Fever is defined as an elevated hypothalamic "set point," whereas exogenous hyperthermia is obtained during passive heating of the body. During hyperthermia the thermoregulatory set point remains unchanged.

An experiment was performed by us to examine whether the increased core body temperature observed during exercise represents a hyperthermic or a prostaglandin-mediated fever reaction. Healthy male volunteers performed bicycle ergometry exercise for 1 hour at 75% of VO_2max. The core body temperature increased linearly to 39.5°C by the end of the experiment. The same experiments

Exercise Immunology, edited by Bente Klarlund Pedersen. © 1997 R.G. Landes Company.

were then repeated at a later day after the subjects had been treated orally with the prostaglandin-inhibitor indomethacin for 2 days. During this treatment the core body temperature did not significantly differ from that of the control experiments (Fig. 4.1). This study lends support to the idea that exercise-induced increases in core body temperature is a hyperthermic reaction and not a prostaglandin-mediated fever reaction. Thus most evidence does not support a change in set point during exercise.[1,2]

Animal studies have demonstrated beneficial effects of hyperthermia and fever in the combat against bacterial and viral

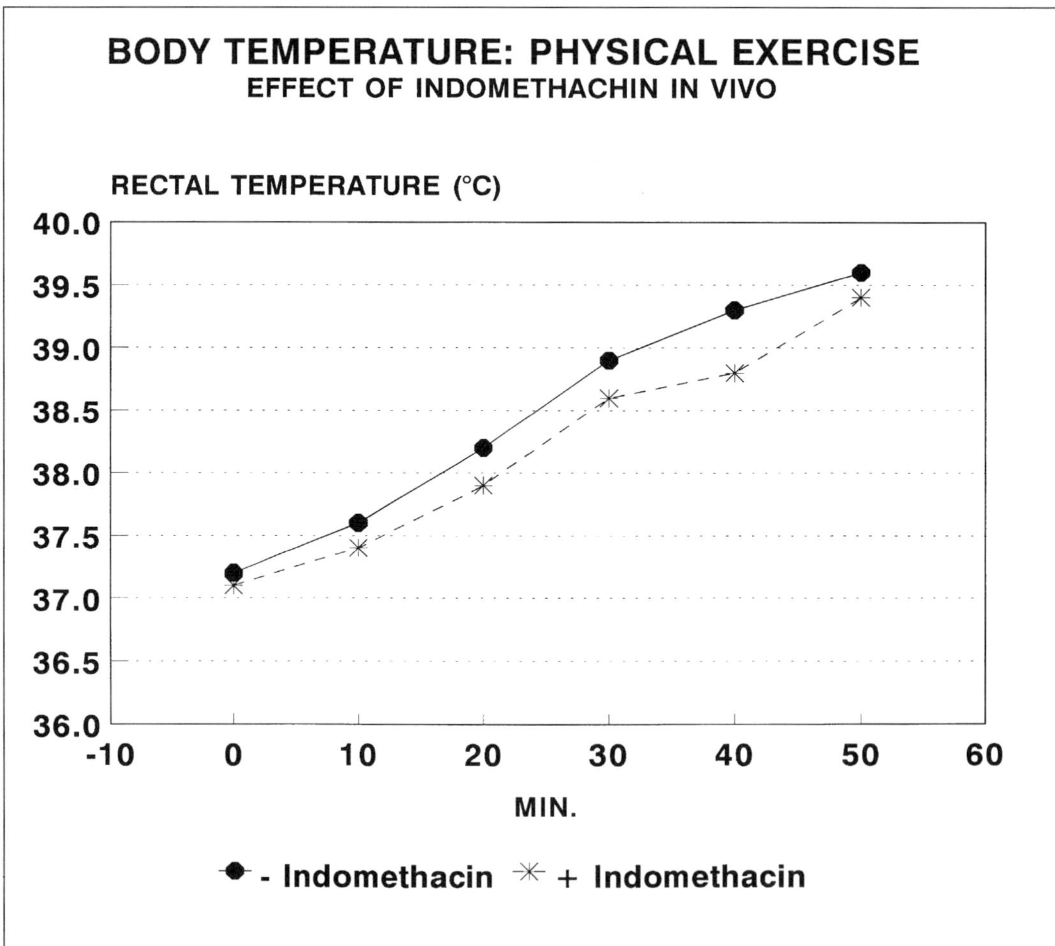

Fig. 4.1. Rectal temperature measured in relation to bicycle exercise 75% VO_2max, 1 hour, with and without treatment with indomethacin. There was no significant difference between the two temperature curves.

infections.[3-6] The in vivo effects of hyperthermia and fever on the immune system have been studied using several models. These include climatic chamber, radio-thermia, heat stroke and water bath.[5] Kappel et al[7-9] studied the influence of in vivo hyperthermia to 39.5°C using a water bath (water temperature 39.5°C). Volunteers were immersed in a water bath for 2 hours, during which their rectal temperature rose to 39.5°C. On a later day they served as their own controls, being immersed into thermoneutral water (34.5°C). The temperature curves are presented in Figure 4.2. This model allowed us to study the isolated effect of increased temperature in humans on the redistribution of lymphocyte subpopulations and cytokine production.

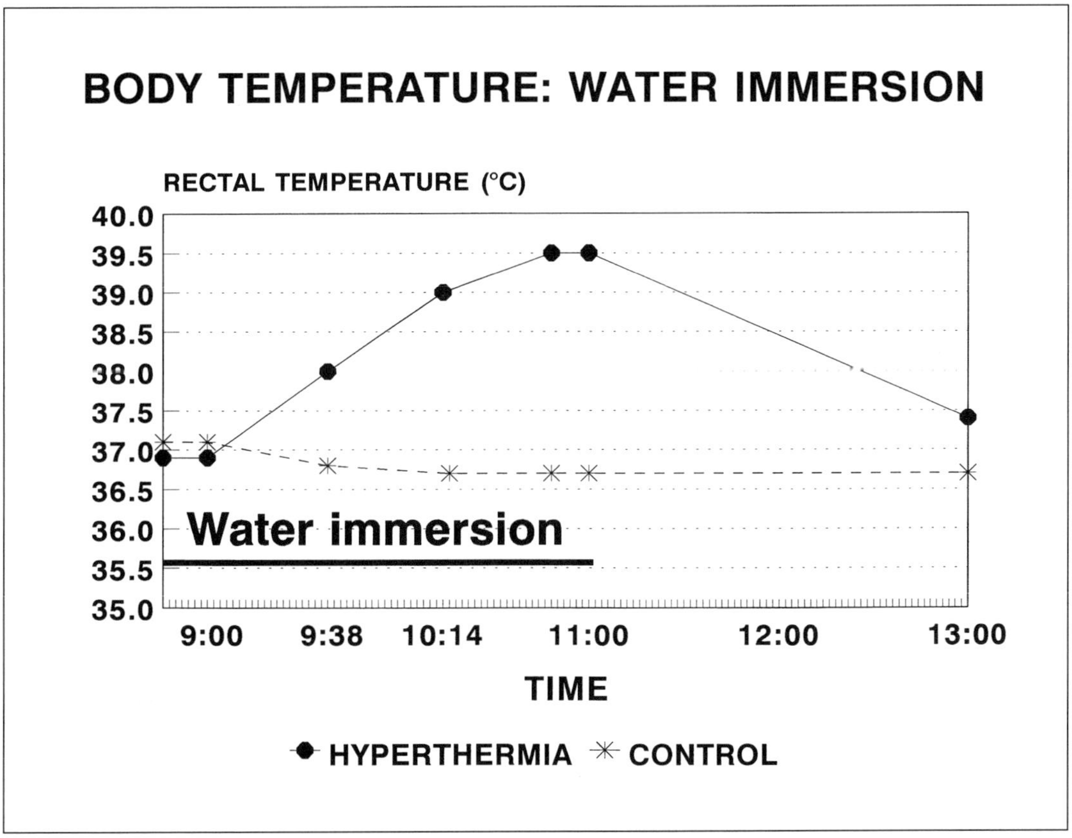

Fig. 4.2. Rectal temperature measured in healthy volunteers immersed into a 39.5°C bath and at thermoneutral conditions. N = 8.

The lymphocyte concentration increased during hyperthermia, predominantly due to an increase in the number of $CD16^+$ natural killer (NK) cells, and the total lymphocyte count was suppressed 2 hours later. The percentage of monocytes did not increase during hyperthermia but increased 2 hours after water immersion. The neutrophil concentration increased during and after hyperthermia (Fig. 4.3).

The NK cell activity increased due to increased proportion of NK cells,[7] but the in vitro proliferative responses to interleukin (IL)-2, phytohemagglutinin (PHA) or purified protein derivative (PPD) did not change.[7] A slight increase in the number of IgM-secreting cells was found 2 hours after water immersion.[10] The numbers of neutrophils and monocytes increased during hyperthermia and were further elevated 2 hours later.[7,8] When the total chemiluminescence and superoxide responses were calculated by multiplying the responses per fixed cell numbers of neutrophils and monocytes with the concentrations of these cells, it was concluded that elevated body temperature caused an increase in the total phagocytic response.

The cytokine-production—IL-1α, IL-1β, tumor necrosis factor (TNF)-α and interferon (IFN)-γ, determined in vitro in lipopolysaccharide or PHA-stimulated blood mononuclear cells (BMNC)—was not influenced by hyperthermia in vivo and the concentrations of plasma-cytokines did not change.[9] In contrast, hyperthermia suppressed the in vitro production of IL-1β, IL-6 and IFN-γ, suggesting that a negative feed-back mechanism does exist between the temperature and the production of some of the molecules involved in the mediation of fever (Fig. 4.4).[11]

Hyperthermia in vitro significantly enhances the in vitro proliferative response of BMNC stimulated with mitogens, antigens or IL-2. Lymphocyte subset analysis before and after incubation with either of these stimulants at 37°C and 39°C showed that hyperthermia increased the proliferation of all cell populations to the same degree (Fig. 4.5).[11] However, in vitro hyperthermia decreased NK cytotoxicity (Fig. 4.6).

The studies by Kappel et al[7-10] are generally in accordance with other studies involving in vivo hyperthermia.[5,12-21] These studies have recently been reviewed by Brenner et al.[5]

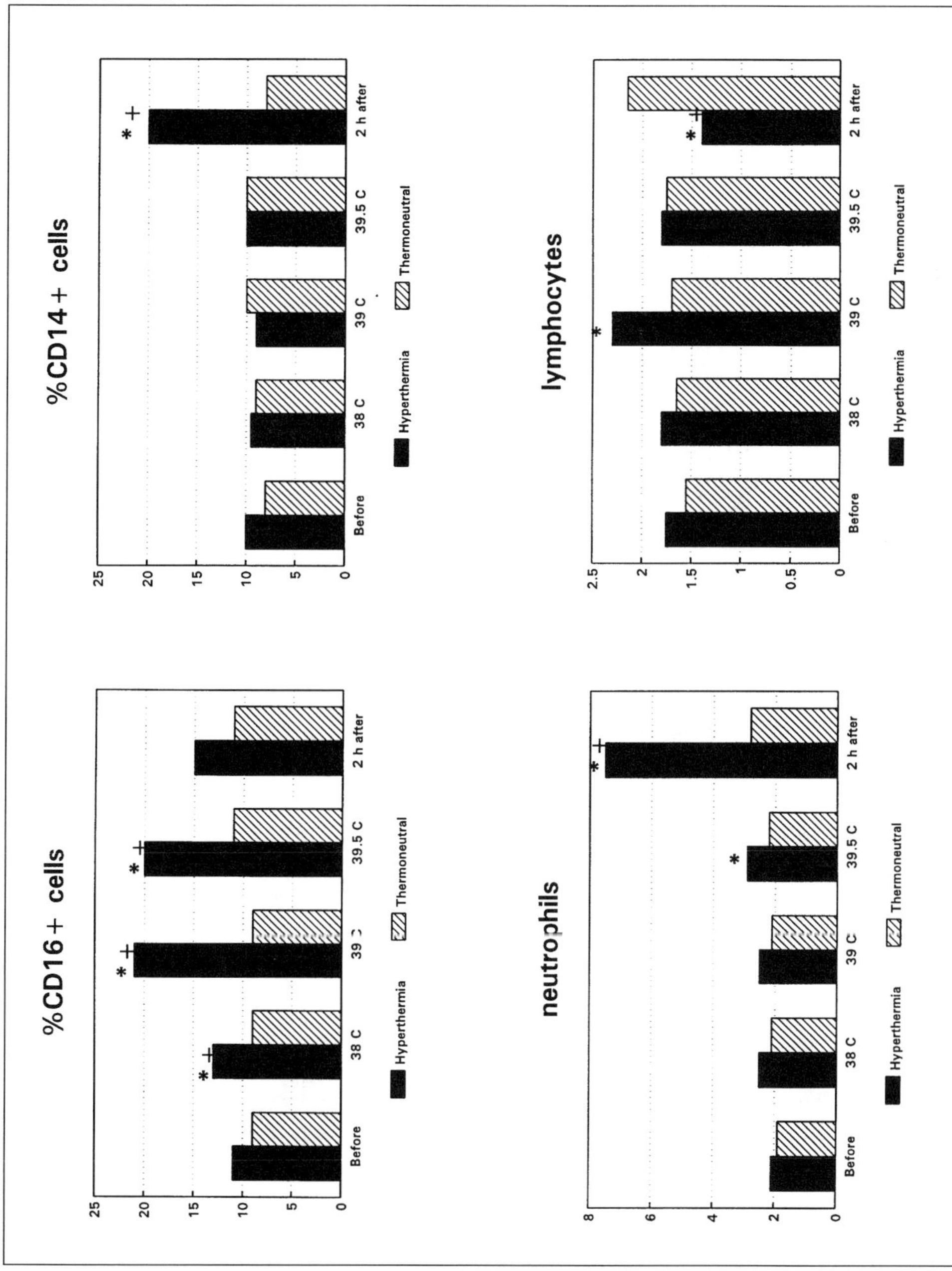

Fig. 4.3. The %CD16+ natural killer (NK) cells, %CD14+ monocytes and concentrations of lymphocytes and neutrophils measured in relation to hyperthermia and control conditions. * denotes significant difference from prevalues, + denotes significant difference between immersion in a hot water bath and thermoneutral water. Results are adapted from Kappel et al.[7]

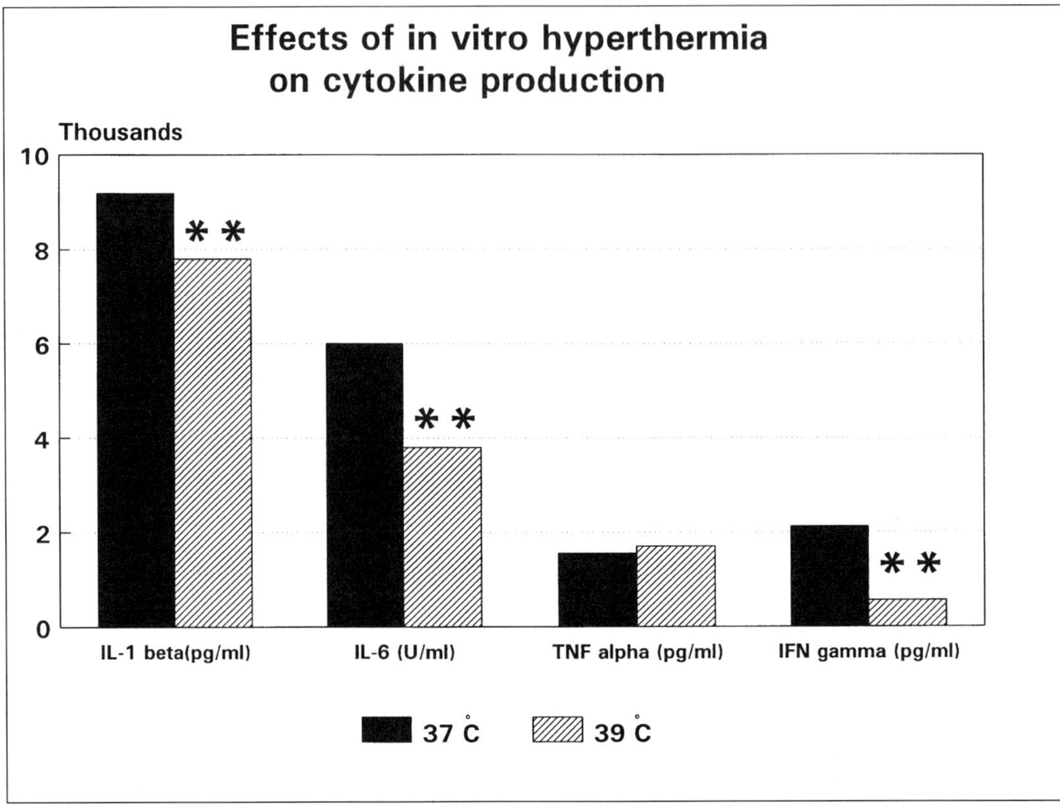

*Fig. 4.4. Effects of in vitro hyperthermia (39°C vs. 37°C) on the production of cytokines from lipopolysaccharide-stimulated blood mononuclear cells. Interleukin(IL)-1β, IL-6, tumor necrosis factor (TNF)-α and interferon (IFN)-γ were measured. ** $p < 0.001$ denotes significant difference between the two temperatures. Results are adapted from Kappel et al.*[11]

The effect of hyperthermia on the recruitment of lymphocytes and neutrophils to the blood resembles the effects of exercise; however, the magnitude of the changes induced by hyperthermia is less than what is generally seen in relation to most exercise models. The neuroendocrinological response induced by hyperthermia differs in many respects from the response seen in exercise.

Hyperthermia induces fewer changes in the concentrations of catecholamines than what is seen in relation to aerobic exercise.[7,22] Thus, although hyperthermia to 39.5°C induced a relative increase (compared to control conditions) in the concentration of catecholamines, the absolute changes were only a 2-fold increase for noradrenaline and less than a 2-fold increase for adrenaline[7] compared

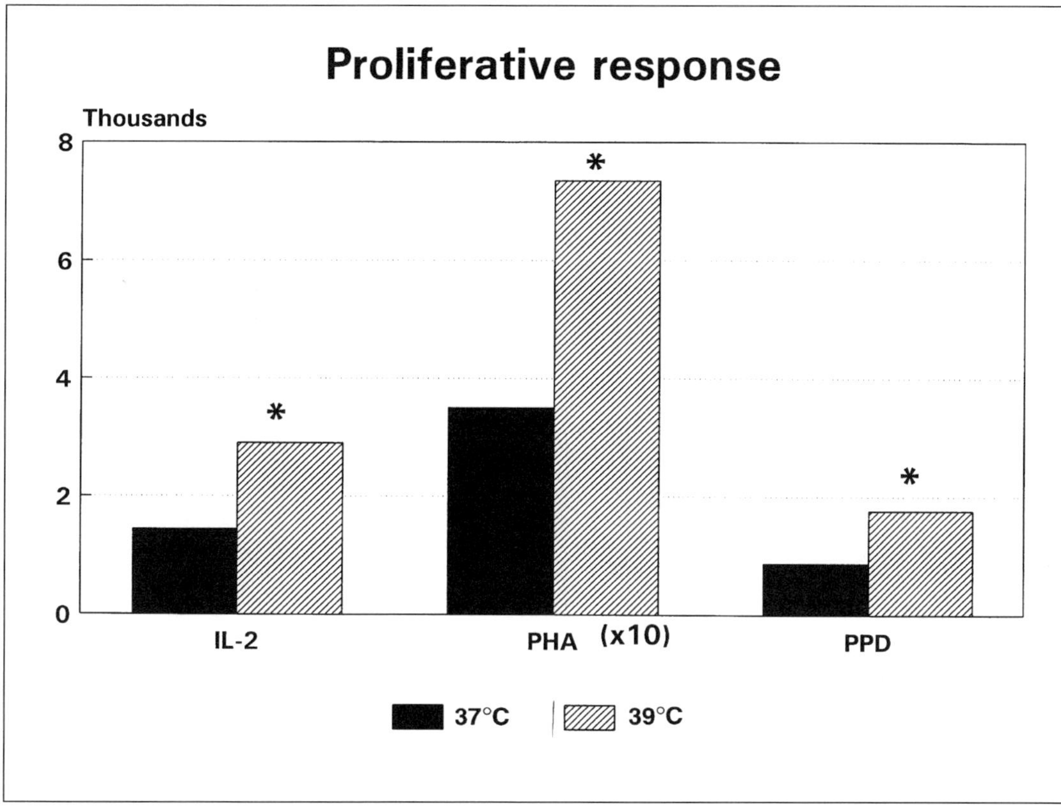

*Fig. 4.5. Effects of in vitro hyperthermia (39°C vs. 37°C) on the proliferative responses following stimulation with interleukin(IL)-2, phytohemagglutinin A (PHA) and purified protein derivative (PPD). * denotes significant difference between the two temperatures. Results are adapted from Kappel et al.[11]*

to eight-fold and 15-fold increases respectively during cycling at 75% of VO_2max for 1 hour.[22] In vivo hyperthermia induced a two-fold increase in the concentrations of cortisol and β-endorphin, resembling that seen during exercise (Kappel et al, manuscript submitted for publication). It appears that serum growth hormone is very sensitive to elevated body temperature. Thus, hyperthermia induced a 25-fold increase in the growth hormone concentration (Kappel et al, manuscript submitted for publication), whereas exercise typically induces a 2-fold peak in serum growth hormone.[23] The concentration in plasma of insulin increases during hyperthermia (Kappel et al, manuscript submitted for publication) and decreases slightly during exercise.[23]

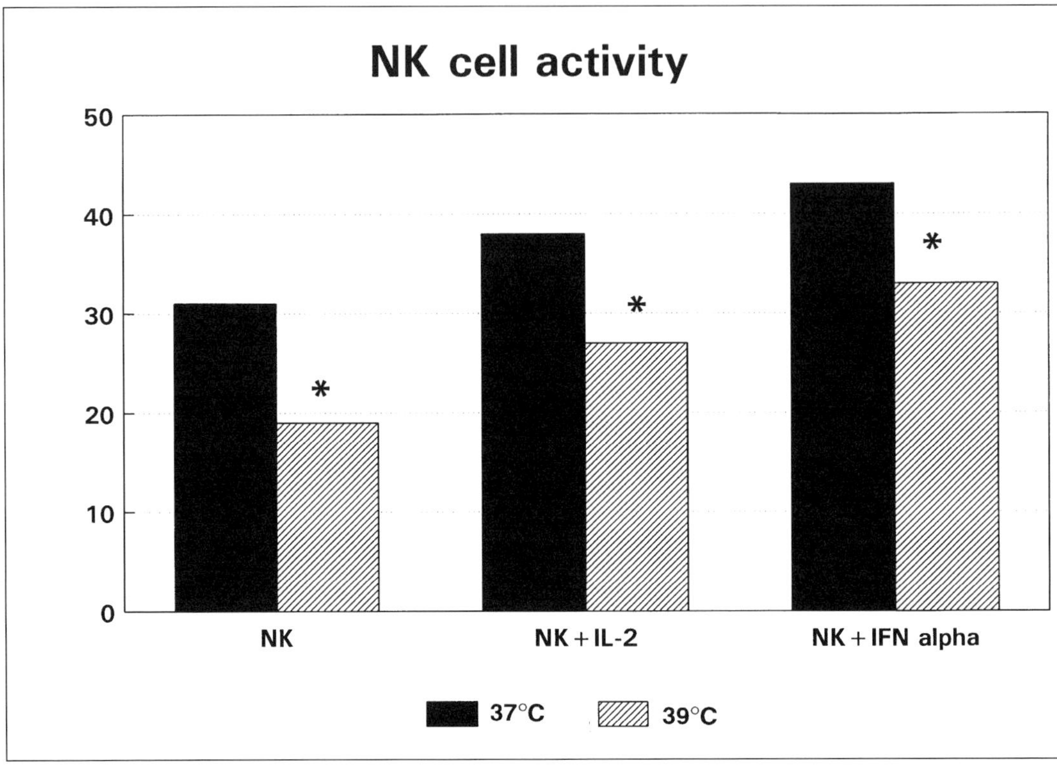

*Fig. 4.6. Effects of in vitro hyperthermia (39°C vs. 37°C) on the natural killer (NK) cell activity. The NK cell activity was measured either unstimulated, and stimulated with interleukin (IL)-2 and interferon (IFN)-α. *denotes significant difference between the two temperatures.*

It is not possible to conclude whether exercise- and hyperthermia-induced immune changes, although comparable, are mediated by the same neuroendocrinological mechanisms.

However, recently, it has been shown that a 2-fold increase in adrenaline concentration during adrenaline infusion (mimicking the effect of hyperthermia) increased the number of NK cells in the circulation, whereas a 2-fold increase in the concentration of noradrenaline had no effect (Kappel et al, manuscript submitted for publication).

Beta-adrenergic blockade inhibited the lymphocytosis during exercise,[24] and during the head-up tilt-induced increase in concentration of NK cells (Klokker et al, manuscript submitted for publication). However, the finding that β-adrenergic blockade during in vivo hyperthermia did not block the increase in NK cell activity indicates that other mechanisms may be responsible for the hyperthermia-associated changes in NK cells (Kappel et al, manuscript submitted for publication). Likewise, blockage of the growth hormone production during hyperthermia by administration of somatostatin partly inhibited the neutrocytosis (Kappel et al, manuscript submitted for publication). These data together with previous results showing that a bolus injection of growth hormone induces neutrocytosis[25] strongly support that the hyperthermia-induced neutrocytosis is partly mediated by growth hormone.

HYPOXIA

Hyperventilation during maximal exercise may counteract the Bohr effect on hemoglobin saturation[26,27] by decreasing alveolar carbon dioxide and increasing alveolar oxygen tensions[28] and, in turn, arterial carbon dioxide ($PaCO_2$) and oxygen (PaO_2) tensions. Yet, PaO_2 and hemoglobin saturation have been reported to be unchanged and even to decrease in well-trained subjects.[29-31] This arterial desaturation may be caused by both a pulmonary diffusion limitation and an effect of pH.

After maximal exercise the diffusion capacity has been shown to decrease.[32,33] Furthermore, "all-out" exercise using several muscle groups as in rowing caused decreased arterial hemoglobin saturation,[34] whereas bicycling and arm cranking did not have this effect. It was shown that arterial hemoglobin saturation decreases in proportion to the muscle mass involved. Since arterial hemoglobin desaturation occurs only during extremely intense exercise involving several muscle groups, it is obvious that arterial desaturation during physical exercise may play no or only a modest role in exercise-induced immunomodulation.

In a study by Klokker et al,[35] in vivo effects of hypoxia on the human immune system were evaluated. Eight young healthy volunteers were placed in a decompression chamber (380 mmHg = 1/2 atm) for 20 minutes with or without supplemental oxygen. Hypoxia caused the leukocyte concentration to increase due to an elevated lymphocyte count. Most notably the $CD16^+$ NK cells increased markedly during hypoxemia, but returned to the pretest value after 2 hours of recovery. Also the NK cell activity of BMNC rose during hypoxia, whereas the absolute concentrations of both $CD8^+$ and $CD14^+$ monocytes increased. Following short term hypoxia the monocyte count decreased again immediately after hypoxia.

In relation to short term hypoxia,[35] the proliferative responses of BMNC after stimulation with PHA, PPD and IL-2 did not change significantly. The in vitro production of IL-1 and IL-2 in supernatants obtained after stimulation with lipopolysaccharide was not affected. The chemiluminescence response of neutrocytes increased 2 hours after hypoxia. It is concluded that acute hypoxia induces marked alterations of the immune system and that NK cells are especially sensitive to hypoxia. Meehan et al[36] found an elevated monocyte concentration during 4 weeks of hypoxia, indicating that chronic hypoxia induces long-lasting adaptations.

In another study,[37] the effect of hypobaric pressure (570 mmHg = 3/4 atm) for 2 hours was investigated. This moderate decrease in environmental pressure increased the neutrocyte concentration but inhibited the chemiluminescence response. The latter finding was confirmed in in vitro studies. Otherwise moderate hypobaric pressure had only minor influence on the cellular immune system of healthy humans.

During exercise the concentrations of all lymphocyte subpopulations became elevated and these responses were enhanced by hypoxia,[38] thus showing the additive effects of two physical stressors, exercise and hypoxia.

CONCLUSION

Exercise is associated with several physiological changes including increased core temperature and in some cases decreased oxygen saturation. The isolated effects of in vivo hyperthermia and hypoxia in humans resemble to some extent the changes observed during exercise. This may be because exercise-, hyperthermia- and hypoxia-induced immune changes are mediated by the same neuroendocrinological mechanisms. However, in vitro studies showing that hyperthermia and hypoxia induce changes in lymphocyte function indicate that physiological alterations during exercise may contribute to exercise-associated immune changes.

References

1. Cannon JG. 3, Exercise and the acute phase response. In: Hoffman-Goetz L, ed. Exercise and Immune Function. New York: CRC Press, 1996:39-54.
2. Stitt JT. Fever versus hyperthermia. Fed Proc 1979; 38:1-10.
3. Bernheim HA, Kluger MJ. Fever: effect of drug-induced antipyresis on survival. Science 1976; 193(4249):237-239.
4. Roberts Jr NJ. Temperature and host defense. Microbiol Rev 1979; 43(2):241-259.
5. Brenner IK, Shek PN, Shephard RJ. Heat exposure and immune function: potential contribution to the exercise response. Exerc Immunol Rev 1995; 1:49-80.
6. Carmichael LE, Barnes FD, Percy DH. Temperature as a factor in resistance of young puppies to canine herpesvirus. J Infect Dis 1969; 120(6):669-678.
7. Kappel M, Stadeager C, Tvede N et al. Effects of in vivo hyperthermia on natural killer cell activity, in vitro proliferative responses and blood mononuclear cell subpopulations. Clin Exp Immunol 1991; 84(1):175-180.
8. Kappel M, Kharazmi A, Nielsen H et al. Modulation of the counts and functions of neutrophils and monocytes under in vivo hyperthermia conditions. Int J Hyperthermia 1994; 10(2):165-173.
9. Kappel M, Tvede N, Hansen MB et al. Cytokine production ex vivo: effect of raised body temperature. Int J Hyperthermia 1995; 11(3):329-335.
10. Kappel M, Barington T, Gyhrs A et al. Influence of elevated body temperature on circulating immunoglobulin-secreting cells. Int J Hyperthermia 1994; 10(5):653-658.
11. Kappel M, Diamant M, Hansen MB et al. Effects of in vitro hyperthermia on the proliferative response of blood mononuclear cell subsets, and detection of interleukins 1 and 6, tumor necrosis factor-alpha and interferon-gamma. Immunology 1991; 73(3): 304-308.
12. Beisel WR, Goldman RF, Joy RJ. Metabolic balance studies during induced hyperthermia in man. J Appl Physiol 1968; 24(1):1-10.
13. Bierman W, Fishberg EH. Some physiologic changes during hyperpyrexia induced by physical means. JAMA 1934; 103: 1354-1357.
14. Bierman HR, Kelly KH, Cordes FL et al. The influence of respiratory movements upon the circulating leukocytes. Blood 1952; 7:533-544.
15. Bull JM, Lees D, Schuette W et al. Whole body hyperthermia: a phase-I trial of a potential adjuvant to chemotherapy. Ann Intern Med 1979; 90(3):317-323.

16. Cohen P, Warren SL. A study of the leukocytosis produced in man by artificial fever. J Clin Invest 1935; 14:423-433.
17. Downing JF, Martinez Valdez H, Elizondo RS et al. Hyperthermia in humans enhances interferon-gamma synthesis and alters the peripheral lymphocyte population. J Interferon Res 1988; 8(2):143-150.
18. Downing JF, Taylor MW, Wei KM et al. In vivo hyperthermia enhances plasma antiviral activity and stimulates peripheral lymphocytes for increased synthesis of interferon-gamma. J Interferon Res 1987; 7(2):185-193.
19. Lakovich VJ. Interferon Res 1988; 8:393-402.
20. Szmigielski S, Sobczynski J, Sokolska G et al. Effects of local prostatic hyperthermia on human NK and T cell function. Int J Hyperthermia. 1991; 7(6):869-880.
21. Ohira Y, Girandola RN, Simpson DR et al. Responses of leukocytes and other hematologic parameters to thermal dehydration. J Appl Physiol 1981; 50(1):38-40.
22. Pedersen BK, Tvede N, Hansen FR et al. Modulation of natural killer cell activity in peripheral blood by physical exercise. Scand J Immunol 1988; 27(6):673-678.
23. Kjaer M, Dela F. Exercise responses to exercise. In: Hoffman-Goetz L, ed. Exercise and Immune Function. New York: CRC Press, 1996:1-20.
24. Ahlborg B, Ahlborg G. Exercise leukocytosis with and without beta-adrenergic blockade. Acta Med Scand 1970; 187:241-246.
25. Kappel M, Hansen MB, Diamant M et al. Effects of an acute bolus growth hormone infusion on the human immune system. Horm Metab Res 1993; 25(11):579-585.
26. Barcroft J. Respiratory Function of the Blood. Cambridge: Cambridge University Press, 1928.
27. Bohr C, Hasselbalch KA, Krogh A. Uber einen biologischer Beziehung wichtigen Einfluss, den die Kohlensuarespannung des Blutes auf dessen Sauerstoffbinding. Skand Arch Physiol 1904; 16:402-412.
28. Klausen K, Secher NH, Clausen JP et al. Central and regional circulatory adaptations to one-leg training. J Appl Physiol 1982; 52(4):976-983.
29. Rowell LB, Taylor HL, Wang Y et al. Saturation af arterial blood with oxygen during maximal exercise. J Appl Physiol 1964; 19:284-286.
30. Holmgren A, Linderholm H. Oxygen and carbon dioxide tensions of arterial blood during heavy and exhaustive exercise. Acta Physiol Scand 1958; 44:203-215.

31. Dempsey JA, Hanson PG, Henderson KS. Exercise-induced arterial hypoxaemia in healthy human subjects at sea level. J Physiol Lond 1984; 355:161-175.
32. Rasmussen BS, Hanel B, Jensen K et al. Decrease in pulmonary diffusion capacity after maximal exercise. J Sports Sci 1986; 4(3):185-188.
33. Hanel B, Clifford PS, Secher NH. Restricted postexercise pulmonary diffusion capacity does not impair maximal transport for O2. J Appl Physiol 1994; 77(5):2408-2412.
34. Rasmussen J, Hanel B, Diamant B et al. Muscle mass effect on arterial desaturation after maximal exercise. Med Sci Sports Exerc 1991; 23(12):1349-1352.
35. Klokker M, Kharazmi A, Galbo H et al. Influence of in vivo hypobaric hypoxia on function of lymphocytes, neutrocytes, natural killer cells, and cytokines. J Appl Physiol 1993; 74(3):1100-1106.
36. Meehan R, Duncan U, Neale L et al. Operation Everest II: alterations in the immune system at high altitudes. J Clin Immunol 1988; 8(5):397-406.
37. Klokker M, Kharazmi A, Galbo H et al. Effects of brief exposure of hypobaric pressure on the immune system. International Review of the Armed Forces Medical Services. 1995; 207-213.
38. Klokker M, Kjaer M, Secher NH et al. Natural killer cell response to exercise in humans: effect of hypoxia and epidural anesthesia. J Appl Physiol 1995; 78(2):709-16.

CHAPTER 5

Exercise, Glutamine and the Immune System

Bente Klarlund Pedersen and Thomas Rohde

Glutamine is the most abundant amino acid in the body. Despite the large number of enzymatic reactions that could cause its depletion, its concentration in the plasma is 500-700 μM and in skeletal muscle 20 mM, thus comprising 50-60% of the free amino acid pool in skeletal muscle. Although glutamine is available in the lumen of the intestine from the digestion of protein, very little of this glutamine enters the blood stream. The absorptive cells of the small intestine utilize glutamine at a high rate and probably utilize almost all that is absorbed from the lumen of the gut.[1]

Hence, to satisfy the high demand for glutamine by various organs, it must be provided within the body. Arteriovenous difference measurements across several tissues indicate that the combined skeletal muscle compartment is by far the most important site for glutamine synthesis. Skeletal muscle has the enzymatic capacity to synthesize glutamine. It contains high activities of branched chain amino acid aminotransferase, glutamine synthetase and other enzymes involved in glutamine metabolism. Glutamine is produced from glutamate and ammonia and catalyzed by glutamine synthetase. Glutamate can be obtained from the circulation, from protein breakdown or from the combination of 2-oxoglutarate and branched chain amino acids (BCAA) (leucine, isoleucine or valine) catalyzed by BCAA transaminase. The

Exercise Immunology, edited by Bente Klarlund Pedersen. © 1997 R.G. Landes Company.

ammonia can be obtained from the free pool of ammonia or donated from the BCAAs via deamination.[2-5] Figure 5.1 shows the major pathways of glutamine production.

GLUTAMINE—A METABOLIC LINK BETWEEN SKELETAL MUSCLE AND THE IMMUNE SYSTEM?

According to Krebs,[6] the reason why such high quantities of glutamine are synthesized is that it has more functions in the body than any other amino acid. Glutamine is required as a nitrogen donor for synthesis of purine and pyrimidine nucleotides and is thereby essential for protein synthesis and cell proliferation.[1-4]

The initial findings in cultured fibroblasts have since been extended to many different cell types, and it is now recognized that glutamine is an important tissue culture supplement necessary for cellular proliferation of a variety of mammalian cells[7-10] including cells of the immune system.[11,12]

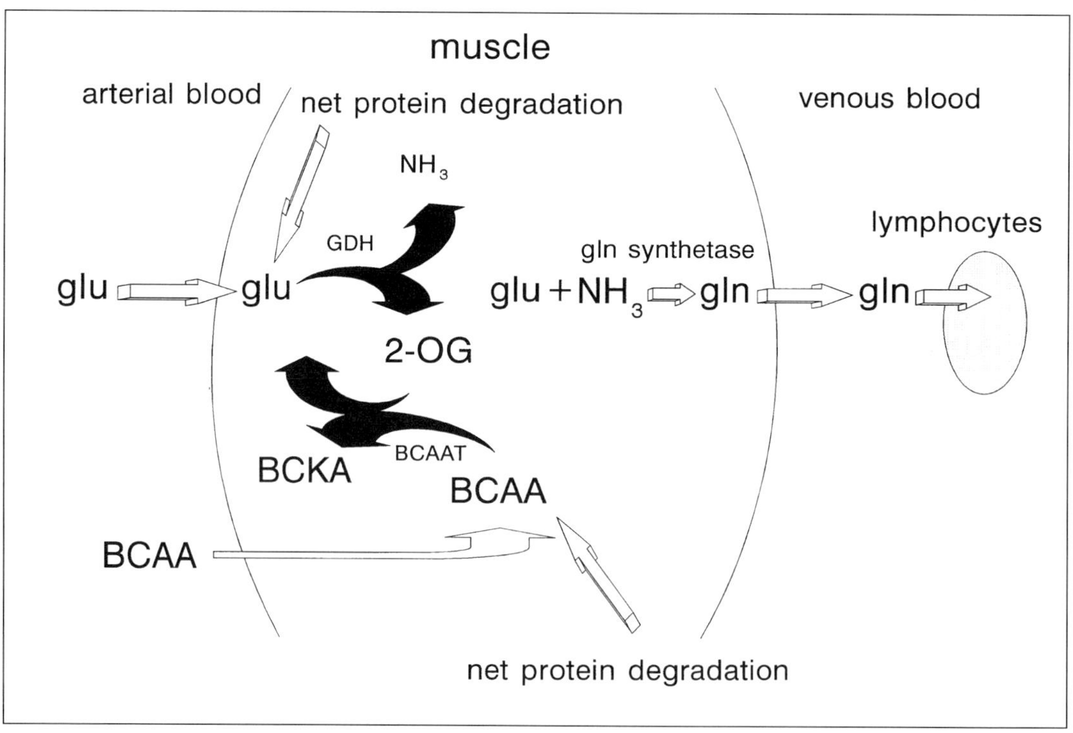

Fig. 5.1 The figure shows the major pathways of glutamine production. glu, glutamate; gln, glutamine; GDH, glutamate dehydogenase; 2-OG, 2-oxoglutarate; BCAA, branched chain amino acids; BCKA, branched chain keto acids; BCAAT, branched chain amino acid transaminase.

It has generally been accepted that cells of the immune system obtain their energy by metabolism of glucose. However, it has been established that glutamine is also an important fuel for lymphocytes and macrophages. Several lines of evidence suggest that glutamine is used at a very high rate by these cells, even when they are quiescent.[2] It has been proposed that the glutamine pathway in lymphocytes may be under external regulation, due partly to the supply of glutamine itself.[13]

As skeletal muscle is the major tissue involved in glutamine production and known to release glutamine into the blood stream at a high rate, it has been suggested that the skeletal muscle plays a vital role in maintenance of the rate of the key process of glutamine utilization in the immune cells. Consequently, the activity of the skeletal muscle may directly influence the immune system. It has been hypothesized (the so called "glutamine hypothesis") that under intense physical exercise, or in relation to surgery, trauma, burn and sepsis, the demands on muscle and other organs for glutamine is such that the lymphoid system may be forced into a glutamine debt, which temporarily suppresses its function. Thus, factors that directly or indirectly influence glutamine synthesis, or release, could theoretically influence the function of lymphocytes and monocytes.[2,14]

LYMPHOCYTE FUNCTION AND GLUTAMINE

The maximal catalytic activities of a number of key enzymes in the metabolism of glutamine—including phosphate-dependent glutaminase—have been measured in lymphocytes and in macrophages, and it has been shown that glutaminase activity is increased during an immunologic challenge (e.g., an infection).[11,15] The initial studies showing a relationship between cell proliferation and the activity of phosphate-dependent glutaminase utilized rat hepatoma cells.[16] The study showed that there was a linear inverse correlation between doubling time and phosphate-dependent glutaminase activity.[16] The increase in glutaminase activity was paralleled by increased activity of various glutamine amidotransferases,[17] decreased intracellular concentrations of glutamine and an increased rate of glutamine consumption.[18] In a manner analogous to the terminology, glycolysis is used to describe partial oxidation of glucose to lactate; the term "glutaminolysis" is used to describe the process of partial glutamine oxidation.[9,19]

The role of glutaminolysis in rapidly dividing cells is to provide both nitrogen and carbon for precursors for synthesis of macromolecules (e.g., purines and pyrimidines for DNA and RNA) and also energy.[20,21] Due to the high rate of glutaminolysis, ideal conditions are present for the control of the use of intermediates for macromolecular synthesis, which is required at a high rate during lymphocyte proliferation in response to an immune stimulus, e.g., an infection. Whereas several studies show that glutamine is essential for cell division of lymphocytes in culture,[15,22] other amino acids, or combinations of glutamate plus ammonia,[15] or glutamate plus leucine,[23] cannot substitute for glutamine.

Macrophage phagocytosis of opsonized antigen has been shown to be glutamine-dependent,[24,25] and the concentration of glutamine has been shown both in humans and animals to be important for the proliferation of lymphocytes, thymocytes, T and B cell lines.[3,11,22,24-28]

The influence of glutamine concentrations on blood mononuclear cell proliferation after stimulation with concanavalin A (ConA), phytohemagglutinin (PHA), purified derivative of tuberculin (PPD) and interleukin (IL)-2 are shown in Figure 5.2.[22] The optimal proliferation was obtained at glutamine concentrations of 0.3-1.0 mM. Similar results were found in another study, showing maximal proliferation with glutamine concentration of 0.3 mM.[11] Flow cytometric analysis showed that several lymphocyte subpopulations are equally dependent on the presence of optimal glutamine in the assay.[22] When the analysis was carried out after the cells had been incubated with either of these agents with or without glutamine, it was shown that the relative fraction of $CD3^+$, $CD4^+$, $CD8^+$, $CD14^+$, $CD16^+$ and $CD19^+$ cells were not changed by glutamine at a concentration of 0.6 mM, except in the PHA-stimulated proliferation experiment where the fraction of $CD4^+$ cells increased. The explanation to the latter is that PHA predominantly stimulates $CD4^+$ cells,[29] and this subpopulation, when stimulated with PHA, is thus more dependent on glutamine.

When blood mononuclear cells (BMNC) were incubated for 48 hours with IL-2 with or without glutamine and tested for

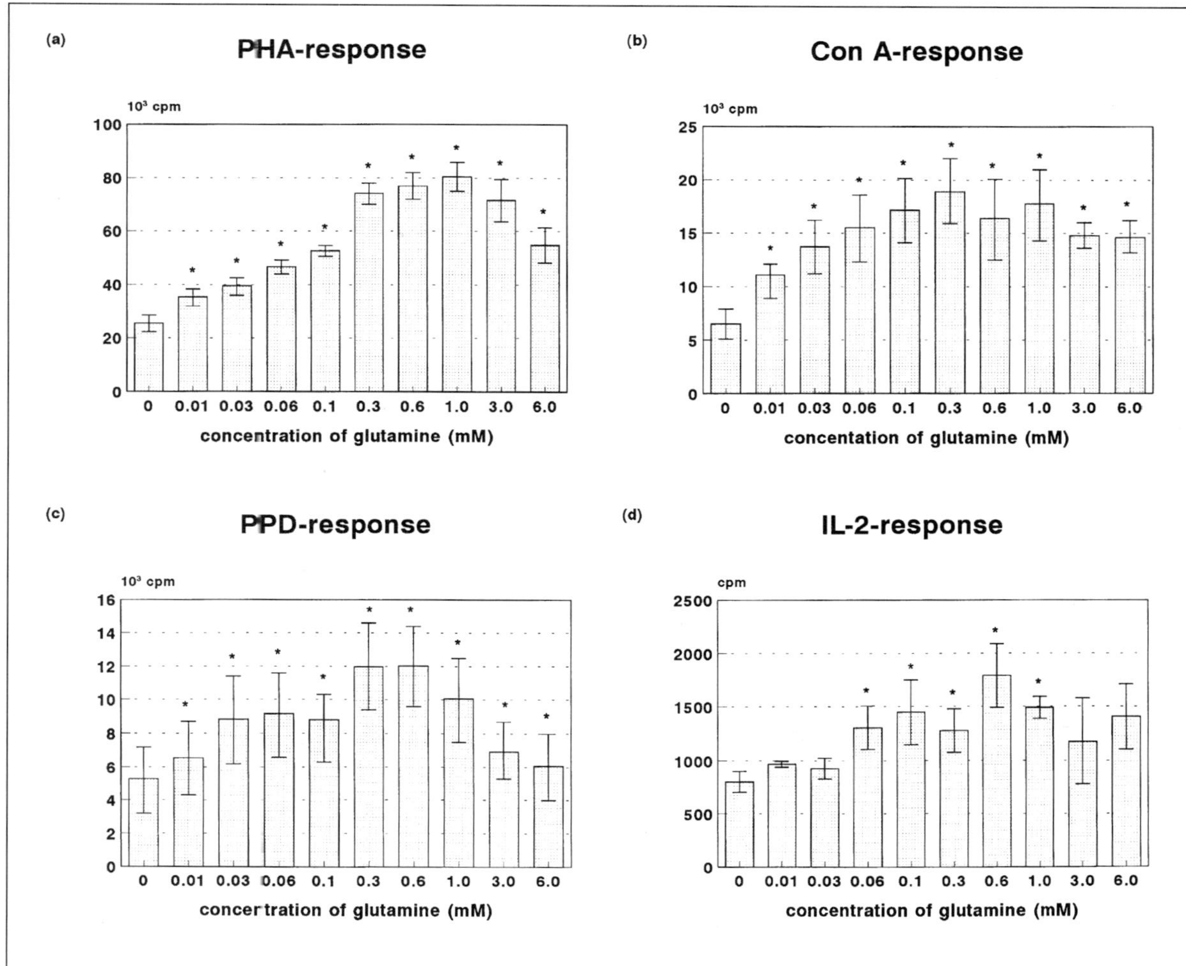

*Fig. 5.2. Proliferative response of blood mononuclear cells incubated with increasing concentrations of glutamine and stimulated with phytohemagglutinin (PHA) (a), concanavalin A (con A) (b), purified protein derivative (PPD)(c), or interleukin (IL)-2 (d). cpm, counts per minute * significant difference from 0 mM glutamine value. Reprinted with permission from Rohde T et al, J Appl Physiol 1995; 79(1): 146-150.*

lymphokine activated killer (LAK) cell activity, the presence of glutamine enhanced LAK cell activity with optimal target cell lysis at a glutamine concentration of 0.3 mM (Fig. 5.3).[22] This was presumably not due to the presence of more LAK cells in the assay, since the percentages of $CD16^+$ or $CD56^+$ cells in the IL-2 proliferation experiments were unaffected by the presence of glutamine. In contrast to the glutamine-LAK cell dependency, the activity of natural killer (NK) cells was not influenced by glutamine.[22] In theory, it was possible that the depressed lymphocyte function in individuals infected with human immunodeficiency virus (HIV) was due to lack of glutamine. However, glutamine supplementation in vitro did not normalize the impaired proliferation of HIV-infected cells. Furthermore, it was shown that glutamine did not abolish the suppressed PHA-response during exercise.[22]

Lymphocyte proliferation is a complex reaction involving a cascade of cytokines. It has recently been shown that glutamine did not influence the production of IL-1β or tumor necrosis factor (TNF)-α, but augmented the production of IL-2, IL-6 and interferon (IFN)-γ. The latter finding explains why glutamine is required for optimal lymphocyte proliferation (Fig. 5.4).[23]

PHYSICAL STRESS, GLUTAMINE AND IMMUNE FUNCTION

Recently, it has been recognized that free glutamine concentrations are very labile under certain physiological conditions. There is an especially marked decline in glutamine concentrations in plasma and body tissues in the presence of catabolic, stressful disease states.[10] During metabolic responses to trauma and sepsis, glutamine is rapidly released by skeletal muscle resulting in decreases in the muscle glutamine concentration.[30-36] Furthermore, following intense longterm exercise and other physical stress disorders, the glutamine concentration in plasma declines. Table 5.1 shows some examples of plasma-glutamine concentrations in relation to exercise, surgery and burns.[3,30,37,38] It should be noted that although plasma glutamine declines in several studies, the lowest concentration measured is still as high as 200 μM (Table 5.1).

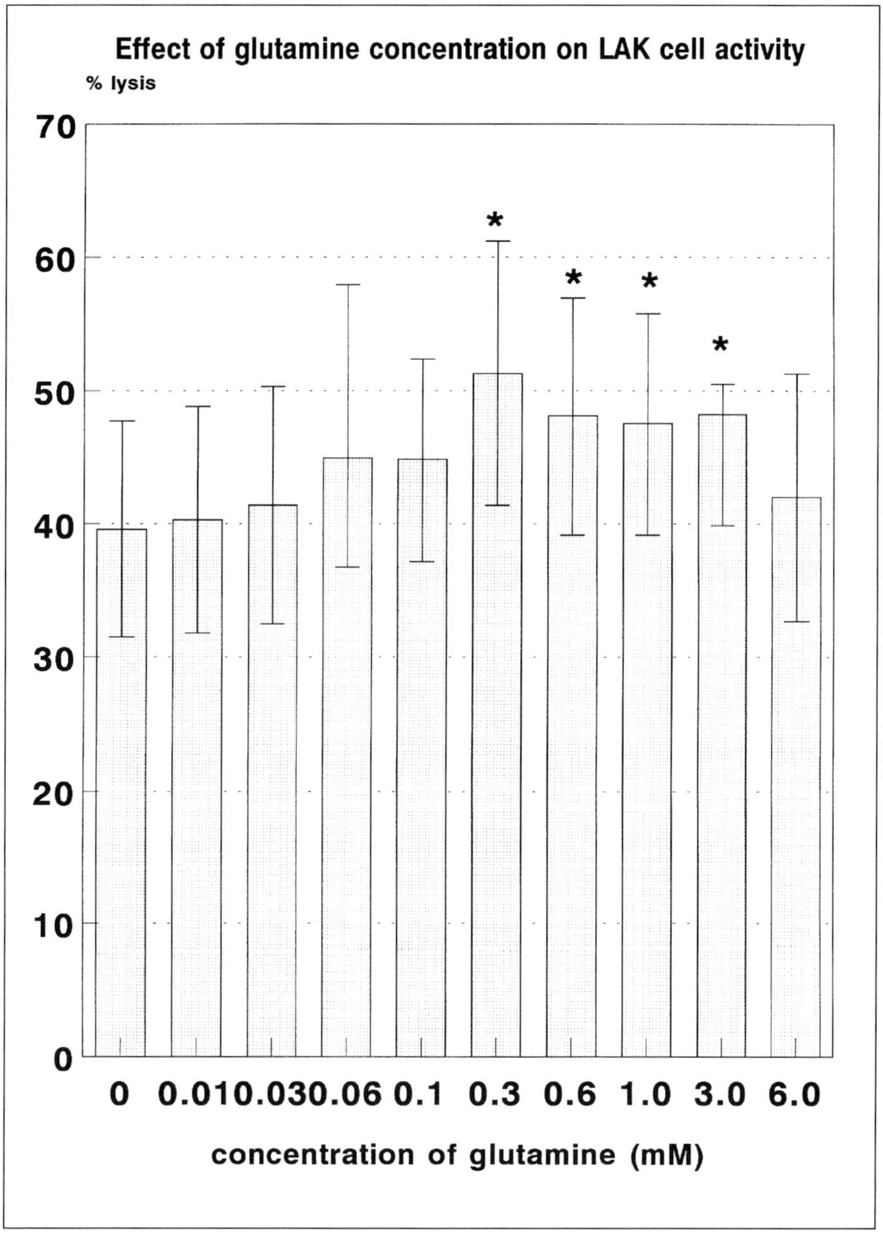

*Fig. 5.3. Effect of glutamine concentration on lymphokine activated killer (LAK) cell activity on blood mononuclear cells incubated with interleukin (IL)-2 for 48 hours and tested for cytotoxicity against Daudi target cells. * significant difference from 0 mM glutamine value. Reprinted with permission from Rohde T et al, J Appl Physiol 1995; 79(1):146-150.*

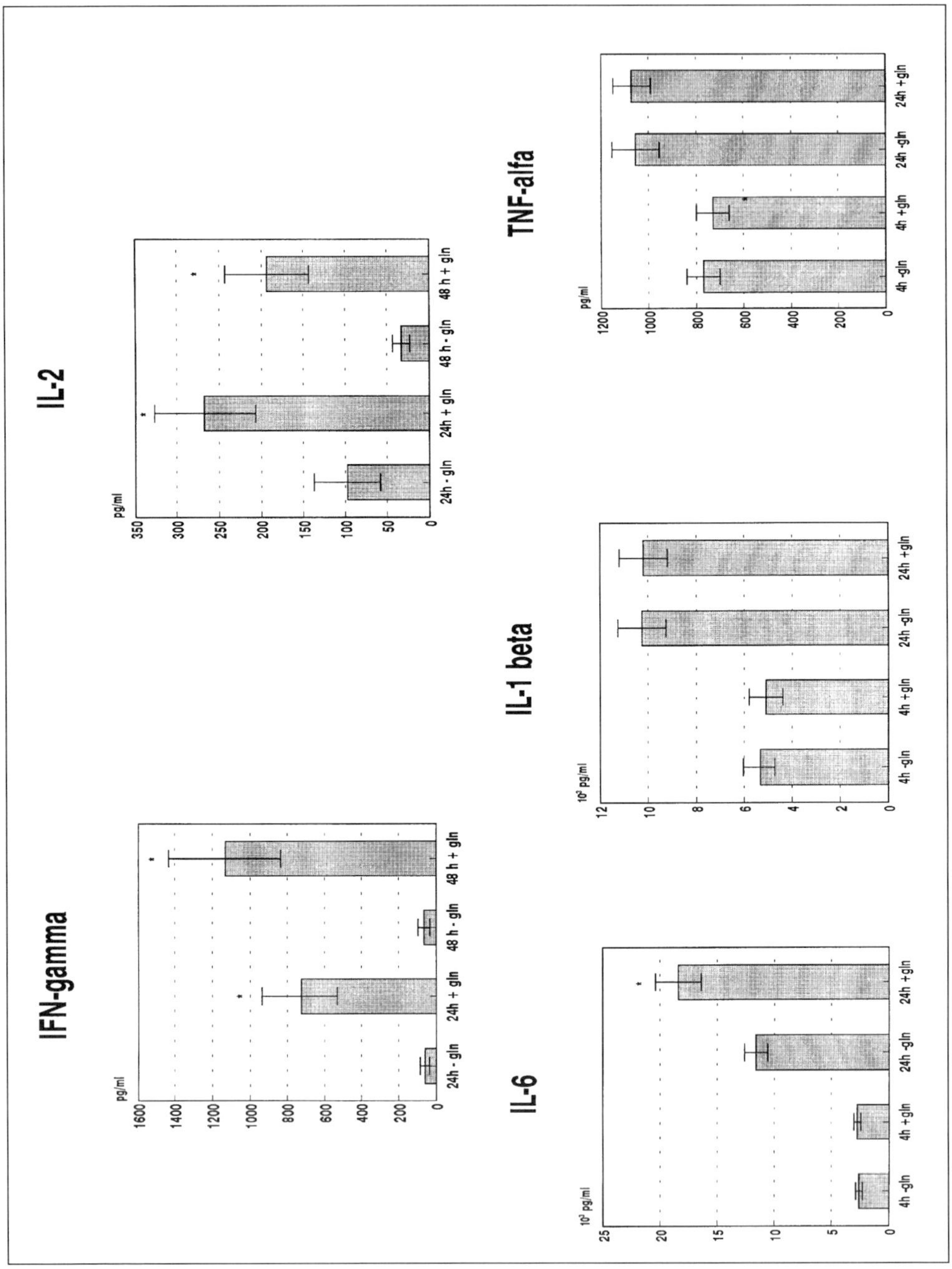

*Fig. 5.4. The effect of glutamine (+gln) on the production of cytokines. Interleukin (IL)-1β, IL-2, IL-6, interferon (IFN)-γ and tumor necrosis factor (TNF)-α. * significant different from controls (-gln). Results are adapted from Rohde et al.*[23]

Table 5.1. Glutamine concentrations in relation to catabolic conditions

Author	Type of Stress	N	gln Conc.μM	gln Conc.μM	P <
Essen[30] 1992	surgical trauma (mean 125 min abdominal surgery)	14	before: 669	24 hrs after: 549	0.001
Keast[37] 1995	15 x 1 min treadmill run (120% VO_2 max)	7	rest: 1244	after (within 5 min): 560	0.01
	Overtraining (10 days of intensive, twice daily interval training)	5	before: 630	day 11: 328	0.08
Lehmann[38] 1995	Ultratriathlon	9	no change		
Parry Billings[3] 1992	overtrained	40	controls: 550	subjects: 503	0.02
	1/2 marathon	24	before: 592	after: 495	0.001
	marathon (+BCAA)	23	before: 581	after: 561	NS
	30 km treadmill run	12	before: 641	after: 694	NS
	cycling (73% VO_2 max)	4	before: 567	after: 615	NS
	sprints (10 x 6s)	10	before: 556	after: 616	0.05
Parry Billings[3] 1992	minor surgery	5	no change		
	major surgery	9	before: 653	48 hrs after.: 455	0.001
Parry Billings[25] 1990	burns (30%)	4	day of burn: 490	11 days after: 200	ND

The acceleration of BCAA metabolism during exercise is paralleled by an increase of the glutamine release from muscle.[4,39] The mechanisms responsible for the decrease in plasma glutamine concentration after longterm exercise and in overtrained athletes is not known. However, Wagenmakers[4] suggests that a reduction in muscle concentration of tricarboxylic acid (TCA) cycle intermediates may lead to a reduction in the synthesis rate of glutamine, or that the synthesis rate of glutamine may fall during exercise due to the fact that the glutamine synthetase reaction is adenosine triphosphate (ATP) dependent.

It has been suggested that decreases in the glutamine pools in relation to the above-mentioned clinical disorders and physical exercise are responsible for the immunosuppression observed in these individuals. However, the weak point in the "glutamine hypothesis" is that if the lowest concentrations of glutamine obtained poststress are added in vitro to the lymphocytes, then these will function as well as at concentrations identical to those obtained at rest.[22]

CONCLUSION

Clearly, optimal lymphocyte proliferation is dependent on the presence of glutamine, but there are no published data showing that glutamine supplementation restores impaired immune function postexercise. The critical question therefore is not whether concomitant decreased plasma-glutamine concentration and lymphocyte function occur following intense exercise, but whether a causal relationship exists. Today, there is no lack of working hypotheses about the functions of glutamine, but there are a lack of experiments to support or reject the hypotheses.

References

1. Windmueller HG, Spaeth AE. J Biol Chem 1974; 49:5070-5071.
2. Newsholme EA. Biochemical mechanisms to explain immunosuppression in well-trained and overtrained athletes. Int J Sports Med 1994; 15:S142-7.
3. Parry Billings M, Budgett R, Koutedakis Y et al. Plasma amino acid concentrations in the overtraining syndrome: possible effects on the immune system. Med Sci Sports Exerc 1992; 24(12):1353-8.

4. Wagenmakers AJM. Amino Acid Metabolism, Muscular Fatigue and Muscle Waisting Speculations on Adaptations at High Altitudes. Int J Sports Med 1992; 13:S110-S113.
5. Bulus N, Cersosimo E, Ghishan F et al. Physiologic importance of glutamine. Metabolism. 1989; 38(8 Suppl 1):1-5.
6. Krebs H. Glutamine metabolism in the animal body. In: Mora J, Palacios R, eds. Glutamine, Metabolism, Enzymology and Regulation. New York: Academic, 1981:319-325.
7. Zielke HR, Ozand PT, Tildon JT et al. Reciprocal regulation of glucose and glutamine utilization by cultured human diploid fibroblasts. J Cell Physiol 1978; 95(1):41-48.
8. Reitzer LJ, Wice BM, Kennell D. Evidence that glutamine, not sugar, is the major energy source for cultured HeLa cells. J Biol Chem 1979; 254(8):2669-2676.
9. McKeehan WL. Glycolysis, glutaminolysis and cell proliferation. Cell Biol Int Rep 1982; 6(7):635-650.
10. Smith RJ. Glutamine metabolism and its physiologic importance. JPEN. J Parenter Enteral Nutr 1990; 14(4 Suppl):40S-44S.
11. Ardawi MS, Newsholme EA. Glutamine metabolism in lymphocytes of the rat. Biochem J 1983; 212(3):835-842.
12. Crawford J, Cohen HJ. The essential role of L-glutamine in lymphocyte differentiation in vitro. J Cell Physiol 1985; 124(2): 275-282.
13. Ardawi MS, Newsholme EA. Intracellular localization and properties of phosphate-dependent glutaminase in rat mesenteric lymph nodes. Biochem J 1984; 217(1):289-296.
14. Newsholme EA. Psychoimmunology and cellular nutrition: an alternative hypothesis [editorial]. Biol Psychiatry 1990; 27(1):1-3.
15. Ardawi MS, Newsholme EA. Maximum activities of some enzymes of glycolysis, the tricarboxylic acid cycle and ketone-body and glutamine utilization pathways in lymphocytes of the rat. Biochem J 1982; 208(3):743-748.
16. Linder Horowitz M, Knox WE, Morris HP. Glutaminase activities and growth rates of rat hepatomas. Cancer Res 1969; 29(6): 1195-1199.
17. Prajda N, Katunuma N, Morris HP et al. Imbalance of purine metabolism in hepatomas of different growth rates as expressed in behavior of glutamine-phosphoribosylpyrophosphate amidotransferase. Cancer Res 1975; 35:3061-3068.
18. Sebolt JS, Weber G. Negative correlation of L-glutamine concentration with proliferation rate in rat hepatomas. Life Sci 1984; 34(3):301-306.
19. Moskovitz B, Katz Y, Singer P et al. Glutamine Metabolism and Utilization: Relevance to major problems in health care. Pharmacol Rev 1994; 30:61-71.

20. Newsholme P, Gordon S, Newsholme EA. Rates of utilization and fates of glucose, glutamine, pyruvate, fatty acids and ketone bodies by mouse macrophages. Biochem J 1987; 242(3):631-636.
21. Larrabee RC. Leucocytosis after violent exercise. The J Med Res 1902; 7:76-82.
22. Rohde T, Ullum H, Palmo J et al. Effects of glutamine on the immune system-influence of muscular exercise and HIV infection. J Appl Physiol 1995; 79(1):146-150.
23. Rohde T, MacLean DA, Pedersen BK. Glutamine, lymphosyte proliferation and cytokine production. Scand J Immunol 1996; (in press).
24. Wallace C, Keast D. Glutamine and macrophage function. Metabolism 1992; 41(9):1016-1020.
25. Parry Billings M, Evans J, Calder PC et al. Does glutamine contribute to immunosuppression after major burns? Lancet 1990; 336(8714):523-525.
26. Ardawi MS. Glutamine and glucose metabolism in human peripheral lymphocytes. Metabolism 1988; 37(1):99-103.
27. Newsholme EA, Parry Billings M. Properties of glutamine release from muscle and its importance for the immune system. J Parenter Enteral Nutr 1990; 14(4 Suppl):63S-67S.
28. Brand K, Fekl W, von Hintzenstern J et al. Metabolism of glutamine in lymphocytes. Metabolism 1989; 38(8 Suppl 1):29-33.
29. Tvede N, Pedersen BK, Hansen FR et al. Effect of physical exercise on blood mononuclear cell subpopulations and in vitro proliferative responses. Scand J Immunol 1989; 29(3):383-389.
30. Essen P, Wernerman J, Sonnenfeld T et al. Free amino acids in plasma and muscle during 24 hours postoperatively—a descriptive study. Clin Physiol 1992; 12(2):163-177.
31. Vinnars E, Bergstom J, Furst P. Influence of the postoperative state on the intracellular free amino acids in human muscle tissue. Ann Surg 1975; 182(6):665-671.
32. Askanazi J, Elwyn DH, Kinney JM et al. Muscle and plasma amino acids after injury: the role of inactivity. Ann Surg 1978; 188(6):797-803.
33. Askanazi J, Michelsen CB, Carpentier YA et al. Sequential changes in muscle and plasma amino acids during injury, infection, and convalescence. Surg Forum 1979; 30:90-92.
34. Askanazi J, Furst P, Michelsen CB et al. Muscle and plasma amino acids after injury: hypocaloric glucose vs. amino acid infusion. Ann Surg 1980; 191(4):465-472.
35. Souba WW, Austgen TR. Interorgan glutamine flow following surgery and infection. J Parenter Enteral Nutr 1990; 14(4 Suppl):90S-93S.

36. Kapadia CR, Colpoys MF, Jiang ZM et al. Maintenance of skeletal muscle intracellular glutamine during standard surgical trauma. J Parenter Enteral Nutr 1985; 9(5):583-589.
37. Keast D, Arstein D, Harper W et al. Depression of plasma glutamine concentration after exercise stress and its possible influence on the immune system. Med J Aust 1995; 162:15-8.
38. Lehmann M, Huonker M, Dimeo F et al. Serum amino acid concentrations in nine athletes before and after the 1993 Colmar ultra triathlon. Int J Sports Med 1995; 16(3):155-159.
39. Eriksson LS, Broberg S, Bjorkman O et al. Ammonia metabolism during exercise in man. Clin Physiol 1985; 5(4):325-336.

CHAPTER 6

Exercise and Cytokines

Bente Klarlund Pedersen, Thomas Rohde and Helle Bruunsgaard

An infection or tissue injury induces a complex cascade of nonspecific events, known as the inflammatory response. The local response involves the production of cytokines which are released at the site of inflammation. These cytokines facilitate an influx of lymphocytes, neutrophils, monocytes and other cells, and these cells participate in the clearance of the antigen and the healing of the tissue. The local inflammatory response is accompanied by a systemic response known as the acute phase response. This response includes increased synthesis of hormones such as hydrocortisone and adrenocorticotropin (ACTH). Furthermore, it includes leukocytosis and the production of a large number of hepatocyte-derived acute phase proteins, e.g., C reactive protein.

The purpose of this chapter is to present evidence for manifestations of an acute phase response following exercise and to discuss whether these manifestations are mechanistically the same as the classical acute phase response. The particular role of cytokines in the acute phase response in relation to exercise will be discussed.

CYTOKINES

Cytokines are a group of regulatory low-molecular weight regulatory proteins secreted by white blood cells and a variety of other cells in the body in response to a number of inducing stimuli. Cytokines generally function as intercellular messenger molecules that evoke particular biological activities after binding to a receptor on a responsive target cell. In the acute phase response, interleukin (IL)-1, IL-6 and tumor necrosis factor (TNF)-α have been most extensively studied.

Interleukin-1 is a name that designates two proteins IL-1α and IL-1β, which recognize the same surface receptors but are the products of distinct genes. Interleukin-1α and IL-1β are structurally related polypeptides that show approximately 25% identity at the amino acid level.

Cells known to produce IL-1 include osteoblasts, monocytes, macrophages, keratinocytes, Kupffer cells, hepatocytes, thymic and salivary gland epithelium, fibroblasts and glial cells. The effects produced by IL-1α and IL-1β result following the binding of these cytokines to two distinct cell surface receptors(R): IL-1R types I and II. In general, type IR binds IL-1α better than IL-1β and the type IIR binds IL-1β more strongly than IL-1α. However, only type IR is capable of transducing a signal and can produce all of the biological effects attributed to IL-1.[1,2]

A naturally occurring inhibitor of IL-1 activity has been described. The molecule is designated interleukin-1 receptor antagonist(IL-1ra).[3-6] Current evidence indicates that the inhibitory action of IL-1ra results from binding of IL-1ra to the receptor type I with an affinity comparable to that of IL-1α or IL-1β, thus competing with IL-1α or IL-1β for binding to this receptor. This binding does not, however, result in signal transduction.[7,8] Thus, IL-1ra exerts its effects by blocking the biological activities of IL-1α and IL-1β and it does not possess independent biological activity.

Cells known to produce IL-1ra include monocytes, neutrophils, macrophages and fibroblasts. Interleukin-6, among other cytokines, has been shown to upregulate IL-1ra.[4-6] Interleukin-6 is expressed by a variety of normal and transformed cells including T cells, B cells, monocytes/macrophages, fibroblasts, hepatocytes, keratinocytes, astrocytes, vascular endothelial cells, mesangial cells and osteoblasts.[9] Interleukin-6 exerts its activity through binding to a high affinity receptor complex consisting of two membrane glycoproteins: an IL-6 binding receptor (IL-6R) and a signal-transducing protein (gp 130).[10] The production of IL-6 is upregulated by IL-1,

IL-2, interferons (IFN) and TNF. Interleukin-6 can induce the synthesis of hepatic acute phase proteins both in vitro and in vivo.

Tumor necrosis factor-α and TNF-β are two closely related proteins that bind to the same cell surface receptors and produce a vast range of similar but not identical effects.[11,12] Tumor necrosis factor-α is produced by neutrophils, activated lymphocytes, macrophages, natural killer (NK) cells, lymphokine activated killer (LAK) cells, astrocytes, endothelial cells, smooth muscle cells and some transformed cells, while TNF-β is produced by lymphocytes.

Two distinct receptor types have been identified that specifically bind TNF-α and TNF-β. Virtually all cell types studied show the presence of one or both of these receptor types designated TNFR-I (55 kDa) or TNFR-II (75 kDa). Each receptor type alone can bind either TNF-α or TNF-β with reasonable high affinity and there is no evidence that interaction between the two receptor types is necessary for signal transduction.[13-16]

There is now evidence that TNFR-1 is probably responsible for the apoptotic effect of TNF-α, whereas TNFR-II is responsible for generating proliferative and regulatory signals in lymphocytes, although this remains to be fully elucidated.[13-16]

Injection of IL-1α, IL-1β, IL-6, TNF-α and TNF-β into laboratory animals[1] or humans[17] will produce most if not all aspects of the acute phase response. These cytokines are therefore usually referred to as "inflammatory or proinflammatory cytokines." Although it has been established that IL-1, IL-6 and TNF play major roles in the pathogenesis of acute and chronic inflammation, their particular role in the acute phase response following exercise is not known.

PLASMA LEVELS OF CYTOKINES IN RESPONSE TO EXERCISE

The first study suggesting that exercise induced a cytokine response was published in 1983 by Cannon and Kluger.[18] They showed that plasma obtained from human subjects after exercise and injected intraperitoneally into rats, elevated rat rectal temperature and depressed plasma iron and zinc concentrations. Plasma obtained prior to exercise failed to produce these responses. The pyrogenic component was heat-denaturable and had an apparent molecular weight of 14,000 Daltons. Human mononuclear leukocytes obtained after exercise and incubated in vitro released a factor into the medium that also elevated body temperature in rats and reduced trace metal concentrations. These results suggested that an endogenous pyrogen was released during exercise.

In 1986, two studies were published on exercise and IL-1[19,20] (Table 6.1). Evans et al[20] studied the effects of 45 minutes eccentric bicycle exercise on IL-1 activity in the plasma in four male runners and five untrained men. Interleukin-1 activity was measured by the ability of Sephadex G-50 chromatographed plasma fractions to increase thymocyte proliferation, and results were expressed as percent basal thymocyte proliferation. Plasma IL-1 activities increased 3 hours after exercise in all five of the untrained men, whereas there was no increase in the trained individuals. Interestingly, the highly trained endurance runners tended to have higher IL-1 activity prior to exercise, but these values did not increase further in response to exercise. Furthermore, the patterns of change in plasma creatine kinase (CK) activities between trained and untrained men were strikingly different. When compared with the trained men, preexercise CK levels were significantly higher in the runners. In the untrained men, CK levels increased progressively for 5 days afterward, reaching a peak value that was 33 times greater than the baseline level. In contrast, the increase in plasma CK level in trained subjects was significant only at 24 hours after the exercise bout, reaching maximum value 2.3 times greater than the preexercise level.

In another study by Cannon et al,[19] IL-1-activity was measured by the thymocyte proliferation bioassay in plasma 3 hours after bicycle exercise for 1 hour. The IL-1 effect was neutralized by an antibody to IL-1. However, although initial findings indicated a correlation between CK and IL-1 levels,[20] this study[19] found no significant correlation between CK level and IL-1 activity in plasma (Table 6.1).

The initial studies thus showed that systemic elevations of cytokines occur in serum after strenuous exercise. The identity of the observed cytokine was, however, uncertain. Recently Bagby et al[21] suggested that although IL-1 was believed to be the cytokine responsible for the exercise-induced plasma activities described by Cannon and Kluger,[18] Cannon et al[19] and Evans et al,[20] the possibility exists that other cytokines were measured. The later studies were conducted prior to the availability of recombinant IL-1 proteins. Furthermore, the thymocyte proliferation bioassay also detects IL-6. Therefore, the possibility exists that the cytokine responsible for the activity measured in the thymocyte bioassay or for the fever-inducing properties of plasma was IL-6 and not IL-1. A number of studies failed to detect significantly elevated levels of IL-1 in plasma (Table 6.1).[22-25]

Northoff and Berg[22] suggested that IL-6 might be involved in the generation of the acute phase response postexercise. They tested 17 participants of a marathon. The serum was tested using the 7TD1 assay, which is very sensitive and specific for IL-6. In 15 of the 17 runners, there was a significant increase of IL-6 measurable immediately after exercise. Using an ELISA kit for IL-1β, they found no detectable IL-1 (Table 6.1).

Ullum et al[23] investigated the effect of concentric exercise on cytokine plasma levels and cytokine pre-mRNA in BMNC. A small (less than 2-fold) but significant increase in plasma IL-6 was found during exercise using an ELISA kit. The plasma levels of IL-1α, IL-1β, IL-6 and TNF-α were below the detection limit in most subjects. Pre-mRNA for IL-1α, IL-1β, IL-6 and TNF-α could be detected in blood mononuclear cells (BMNC) using nuclear run-off analysis, but the amounts did not change in relation to exercise. The same results were obtained when run-off analysis was performed on BMNC after incubation for 2 hours at 37°C and on BMNC isolated at various time points in relation to exercise (Table 6.1).

Several studies have failed to detect TNFα after exercise.[23,26-28] However, Dufaux and Order[29] and Espersen et al[30] reported increased plasma TNFα concentrations 2 hours after completing a 2.5 hours running test or a 5 km race. The disparity between the studies may be explained by the fact that the two later studies[29,30] investigated the cytokine response in relation to eccentric exercise, whereas the former studies[23,26-28] investigated concentric exercise (Table 6.1).

The effect of exercise on plasma interferon (IFN) activity was studied in eight male subjects before and after bicycle exercise for 1 hour. IFN-α increased immediately and 1 hour after exercise.[31]

Table 6.1. Inflammatory cytokines in plasma/serum in relation to exercise

Author	Exercise Type	Modification	N	Time	IL-1β	IL-6	TNF-α	Method
Evans[20] 1986	45 min eccentric	untrained trained runners	5 4	3 h post	↑ ⇔			Thymocyte assay
Cannon[19] 1986	1 h, 60%VO_2 max		8	6 h post	↑			Bioassay
Cannon[25] 1991	45 min eccentric	vit. E suppl. placebo	8 10	6 h post 6 h post	⇔ ↗	UD UD	⇔ ⇔	RIA
Rivier[26] 1994	Incremental max test		10	during, 20 min post			UD	immunoassay
Northoff[22] 1991	Marathon		17	end exercise	↑	↑		Elisa, 7TD1-assay
Rohde* 1996		Marathon	8	during, 2 h post	UD	⇔	UD	Elisa
Rohde* 1996	1h eccentric		6	2 h post	UD	↑	UD	Elisa
Smith[27] 1992	1h cycling, 60%VO_2 max	8 trained and 8 untrained	16	End of exercise 3 h post 6 h post	↗ ↗ ↗	⇔ ⇔ ⇔	↗ ↗ ↗	RIA

Espersen[30] 1990	5 km race	Runners	11	End of exercise			⇔	RIA
				2 h post			↑	
				24 h post			⇔	
Ullum[23] 1994	1h cycling, 75%VO_2 max		17	End of exercise	UD	↑	UD	ELISA
				2 h post	UD	⇔	UD	
Sprenger[24] 1992	20 km race	Runners	22	End of exercise	UD	↑	UD	ELISA
				2 h post	UD	↑	UD	
				3 h post	UD	↑	UD	
				7 h post	UD	↑	UD	
				24 h post	UD	⇔	UD	
Bruunsgaard* 1995	30 min eccentric	Middle-trained	9	End of exercise	UD	↗	UD	ELISA
				2 h post	UD	↑	UD	
				48 h post	UD	⇔	UD	
	30 min, 65% VO_2 max	Same group as above		End of exercise	UD	⇔	UD	
				2 h post	UD	⇔	UD	
				48 h post	UD	⇔	UD	

↑ Significant difference from pre-exercise value
↗ Trend
⇔ No significant difference from pre-exercise value
UD undetectable
** Unpublished data

The plasma IL-2 concentration decreased immediately after a 5 km race.[30] To date, this is the only cytokine reported to decrease in relation to exercise.

Increased cytokine levels after exercise have been found mainly in relation to eccentric exercise or combinations of eccentric and concentric exercise. Helle Bruunsgaard et al[32] performed a study to test the hypothesis that the exercise-induced increase in cytokine levels was associated with muscle damage. Healthy young males performed two bouts of bicycle exercise, the first trial consisted of 30 minutes concentric, whereas the second consisted of 30 minutes eccentric exercise. The CK level increased almost 50-fold 4 days after eccentric exercise, whereas there was no changes in CK level in relation to concentric exercise. The IL-6 level increased 5-fold in relation to eccentric exercise, but was unchanged in relation to concentric exercise. Thus, the study supports the hypothesis that the postexercise cytokine production is related to skeletal muscle damage.

Thus, IL-6 have been described to be enhanced in a number of studies.[22-24] Although increased IL-6 production has been described primarily in relation to eccentric exercise, no studies have shown a significant correlation between CK or other measures of muscle damage and concentration of IL-6 in plasma.

URINARY CYTOKINE RESPONSES TO EXERCISE

Sprenger et al[24] examined the cytokine production in a group of 22 well-trained runners covering a distance of 20 km within 2 hours. Cytokine production was measured in the urine over the subsequent 24 hours. Except for IL-6, other cytokines could not be reliably detected in plasma at all time points studied. In contrast, cytokines could be reproducible determined in urine. Directly after running, a significantly enhanced IFN-γ content was found in the urine of all participants. One hour later, IFN-γ secretion had markedly declined. Tumor necrosis factor-α content in urine peaked directly after finishing the run. One hour later, TNF-α still remained elevated, but thereafter TNF-α values declined. In contrast to IFN-γ and TNF-α, running induced a high and persistent increase of IL-1β excretion into the urine. Directly after exercise, the IL-1β content was not essentially different from preexercise levels, but 1 hour later, high concentrations of IL-1β were found which remained elevated until the next day. Unlike IL-1β, excretion of IL-6 into urine occurred rapidly after exercise and remained elevated up to 7 hours. Interleukin-6 was the only cytokine which could be reliably measured in plasma where it increased directly after running and remained detectable during the following 7 hours. Soluble IL-2receptor (IL-2R) levels in urine increased rapidly directly after running but excretion came to an abrupt end 1 hour later. Sprenger et al[24] also found that IFN-γ, IL-1β, TNF-α and IL-6 values were chronically elevated in the urine of trained versus untrained individuals.

The study by Sprenger et al[24] clearly shows that the cytokine cascade is activated as a consequence of exercise. It is interesting that although exercise has a minimal effect on most circulating cytokine values, several cytokines can be measured in the urine. This indicates that some cytokines are produced, but rapidly removed from the circulation, in response to exercise. Thus, although most studies fail to detect circulating cytokines other than IL-6 in the plasma, the presence of multiple cytokines in urine following exercise indicates that exercise may alter the local production of several cytokines and these may have important paracrine functions.

LPS- AND MITOGEN-INDUCED CYTOKINE PRODUCTION IN RESPONSE TO EXERCISE

A handful of studies have described the in vitro production of cytokines from BMNC, either unstimulated or stimulated with mitogens or lipopolysaccharide (LPS).[25,33-36] Haahr et al[33] examined the effect of concentric bicycle exercise for 1 hour at 75% of VO_2max on the in vitro production of IL-1α, IL-1β, IL-6, TNFα, IL-2 and IFNγ. The production of IL-1α, IL-1β and IL-6 increased significantly after exercise compared to prevalues, whereas the production of TNFα, IL-2 and IFNγ did not change. The increased in vitro production of IL-1β and IL-6 in the supernatants from a fixed number of LPS-stimulated BMNC after exercise was most likely explained by the increased percentage of $CD14^+$ monocytes. Interleukin-2 and IFNγ are both mainly produced by $CD4^+$ and $CD16^+$ cells. During exercise the percentage of $CD4^+$ cells decreases and the percentage of $CD16^+$ cells increases. The findings of unchanged production of IL-2 and IFNγ could therefore be expected. These findings together with the finding that supernatants from unstimulated BMNC did not contain any cytokines indicate that the monocytes are not activated in response to concentric exercise.

Lewicki et al[34] studied trained male endurance bicycle racers, who performed a maximal bicycle test to exhaustion. The in vitro IL-1 production was increased immediately and 2 hours after in accordance with the findings by others.[25,33]

Cannon et al[25] performed a double-blind placebo-controlled study. They examined the effect of vitamin E supplementation for 48 hours on the exercise-induced acute phase response. The volunteers were either young (average age 25 years) or elderly (average age 65 years) sedentary men. They performed 45 minutes of eccentric exercise (downhill treadmill). Twenty-four hours after this single session of eccentric exercise, endotoxin-induced secretion of IL-1β was augmented in cells obtained from the placebo subjects, but no significant changes were observed in cells from the vitamin E-supplemented subjects. In contrast, in this study IL-6 secretion did not increase after exercise, but vitamin E supplementation reduced IL-6 secretion throughout the 12 day period of observation.

The finding by Cannon et al[25] that the IL-1β and the TNFα secretion was increased the morning after exercise without any current changes in mononuclear cell numbers indicate that the monocytes are activated in relation to eccentric exercise.

The effect of vitamin E on IL-1β and IL-6 could not be ascribed to changes in PGE_2[25]. Oxygen radicals enhance endotoxin-induced IL-1.[37] Furthermore, the concentration of these reactants increase with exercise.[38] Thus, the effects of vitamin E on the secretion of IL-1β is consistent with a mechanism involving oxygen radicals.

The results have been inconsistent regarding the in vitro production of TNFα following LPS-stimulation of human BMNC or whole blood. Thus, Kvernmo et al[35] and Northoff and Berg[36] reported decreased TNFα levels after 30 km cross country ski respectively after a marathon race. Haahr et al[33] reported that there was no change after 1 hour of bicycle exercise, and Cannon et al[25] found increased production after 45 minutes of eccentric exercise.

Bagby et al[21,39] reported that the in vivo LPS-induced TNFα response was suppressed in rats after exercise to exhaustion. In these experiments, rats were exercised to near exhaustion. At the completion of exercise, rats were administered LPS intravenously. Exercise had a dramatic effect on the in vivo production of TNFα. Thus, the plasma TNFα response was suppressed by more than 90% with exercise. Future studies will hopefully identify the endogenous mediators responsible for the exercise-induced suppression of the in vivo LPS-induced TNFα production.

ENDOTOXEMIA IN EXERCISE

The mechanisms underlying the enhanced plasma-cytokine level after eccentric exercise still remain unknown. In a recent review, Camus et al[40] describe that strenuous exercise is accompanied by an acute inflammatory response having some similarities with those observed in pathological states, such as trauma and sepsis with Gram-negative bacteria. While the role of LPS endotoxin is undeniable in triggering the septic disease, its possible role in exercise is based on only a few studies.

LPS is a cell wall constituent of Gram-negative bacteria and it is present in the colon at very high levels. When endotoxin enters into systemic circulation, it triggers a cascade of cytokines involving IL-1β, IL-6 and TNFα. These cytokines mediate the sepsis syndrome. Heat stroke is somewhat similar to the sepsis syndrome in that it involves elevations of serum endotoxin, IL-1 and TNFα.[41]

For systemic endotoxemia to occur, the mechanical barrier of the bowel wall, the immunologic barrier of the gut-associated lymphatic tissue and the filtering capacity of the liver must all be overcome. It has been demonstrated that during heat stroke, endotoxin enters the blood as a consequence of intestinal ischemia.[42] Endotoxins may also be released from the ischemic gut into the circulation during exhaustive running when blood flow is diverted away from the splanchnic circulation to exercising muscle.

Brock-Utne et al[43] measured plasma levels of LPS endotoxin and anti-endotoxin IgG in 89 randomly selected, exhausted runners after an 89.4 km road race. They found that 81% of these athletes had plasma endotoxin concentrations above the upper limit of 0.1 ng/ml, including 2% with plasma levels above 1 ng/ml, a value which is considered to be lethal in humans. Interestingly, these authors noticed that the highest endotoxin values were measured in the least fit subjects who completed the race in more than 8 hours. Furthermore, they described a negative correlation between plasma endotoxin and anti-endotoxin IgG values measured after the race. Plasma LPS concentration had returned to normal 1-3 weeks later; 80% of the runners examined during this postexercise period had increased anti-endotoxin IgG concentration.

Rosenberg et al[44] found an increase in the plasma levels of LPS in athletes who took part in a triathlon competition. Three weeks after the 89.4 km road race, Brock-Utne et al[43] studied the effects of a 21.1 km run on plasma LPS levels. They did not find any increase in LPS levels in the participants in this run. According to these authors, it is possible that the absence of an exercise-induced rise in LPS concentration could be due to that the anti-LPS IgG in these individuals could bind circulating endotoxin and facilitate its clearance by the reticulo-endothelial system. Thereby, a relatively mild endotoxemia could be masked.

In the study on exhausted ultramarathon runners,[43] 81% of runners who had plasma endotoxemia in excess of 100 pg/ml had nausea, vomiting or diarrhea. In contrast, only 18% of runners who had plasma endotoxemia levels less than 100 pg/ml suffered from these symptoms. Moore et al[45] studied the relationship between mild post-exertional illness in 39 cyclists after a 100-mile ride and found that endotoxemia was not the cause of post-exertional illness and unrelated to rhabdomyolysis. The disparity between the studies on runners[43] and cyclists[45] regarding endotoxemia-associated illness is not easily understood. It is, however, possible that gut trauma during running, but not during cycling, may compromise the barrier function of the bowel wall and thereby increase the portal burden of endotoxins.

It remains to be shown that systemic endotoxemia is the cause of elevated levels of cytokines in the plasma. If so, it would be expected that the cytokines were produced by monocytes in the blood in response to exercise. This has not been shown. The finding by Ullum et al[23] that exercise did not induce changes in BMNC mRNA for proinflammatory cytokines indicate that the cytokines are not of blood origin. However, it cannot be excluded that we were unable to find changes in mRNA due to insensitivity of the run-off analysis and due to the fact that a concentric model was used which gave rise to only a small increase in IL-6.

INITIAL MUSCLE DAMAGE IN EXERCISE—ROLE OF CYTOKINES

Increased cytokine level after exercise is primarily found after exercise associated with muscle damage. The critical question is, whether a causal relationship exists, i.e., does muscle damage cause cytokine production or vice versa?

An eccentric muscle activation is the controlled lengthening of the muscle under tension. In the 1950s, Asmussen[46] established that it was predominantly eccentric as opposed to concentric or isometric muscle action that caused sensation of delayed onset muscle soreness. It is now well recognized that eccentric contractions are more likely than concentric contractions to cause muscle damage.[47,48]

Unaccustomed eccentric muscle action results in disruption of contractile tissue and there also appears to be disruption of connective tissue elements.[49] The sensation of muscle pain appears to be related to this muscle and/or connective tissue disruption. What remains controversial is the association between tissue injury initiated during the exercise bout and the soreness first experienced 24 hours after the exercise.[50]

Several researchers agree that some aspects of an inflammatory reaction is seen in relation to eccentric exercise.[20,49,51-54] The cellular phase of inflammation involves predominantly two types of white blood cells, neutrophils and monocytes. Within a few hours after tissue injury there is a dramatic increase in the number of circulating neutrophils, soon thereafter the cells begin to concentrate at the site of disruption. The neutrophil concentration in the damaged muscle peaks between 1 and 4 hours after the injury and then declines rapidly. Monocyte migration begins several hours after neutrophil migration.

Exercise physiologists have been intrigued by the phenomenon of delay between the initiation of the injury and the onset of soreness 24 hours later. The generation of painful sensation involves activation of pain afferents. In addition certain chemical substances such as prostaglandins of the E series are also required.

Increased levels of PGE_2 and delayed onset muscle soreness have been found 24 hours after a bout of eccentric exercise. The time course for PGE_2 and muscle pain indicates a possible relationship. The source of prostaglandin production could be the macrophages, which is the predominant cell type at 24 hours. However, what is the stimulus for PGE_2 release? Both IL-1α, IL-1β and TNFα have been shown to induce prostaglandin synthesis in endothelial cells, macrophages, smooth muscle cells and skeletal muscle.[1,55-58] Therefore, the production of inflammatory cytokines in response to exercise may stimulate the production of prostaglandins. Further support of this theory is the fact that the high levels of especially plasma IL-6 is found immediately after the completion of an exhaustive exercise. Thus, the IL-6 production or release precedes neutrophil and macrophage accumulation in the muscle, the increase in PGE_2, the increase in CK and the sensation of delayed onset muscle soreness.

However, the interactions between cytokine production and prostaglandins seem to be highly complex. A recent study showed inhibitory effects of PGE_2 on TNF-α and IL-6 production by LPS-stimulated macrophages. The authors suggested that the anti-inflammatory effect of PGE_2 on mononuclear phagocytes is mediated in part by an autocrine feedback mechanism involving IL-10.[59] Interpretation of these results in the acute phase response in exercise make us suggest that PGE_2 exerts a negative feedback mechanism on the cytokine response, whereby the inflammatory response in the muscle is limited.

If the prostaglandins are locally produced from monocytes or macrophages in the muscle, it is most likely that the cytokines are also locally produced. Macrophages and monocytes are the primary source of inflammatory cytokines. Although muscles have few macrophages immediately after exercise, these cells are such potent cytokine producers that only few cells would be required. Alternatively, neutrophils or vascular endothelial cells may be responsible for the production of cytokines.

The time course of cytokine production and the finding that eccentric more than concentric exercise induces a cytokine response strongly indicate the following: during eccentric exercise, myofibers are mechanically damaged and this process stimulates the production of inflammatory cytokines.

PROLONGED MUSCLE DAMAGE AND PROTEIN BREAKDOWN IN EXERCISE—ROLE OF CYTOKINES

Although the cytokines are probably produced in response to the initial mechanical muscle damage, they may play a role in prolonged muscle damage and protein breakdown. Ryan and Majno[60] state, "It is now well established that the inflammatory reaction—although it represents, typically, a reaction to damage—can bring about some local damage of its own." Smith[61] discusses neutrophils and inflammation as "the double-edged sword" by stating, "Although destruction of infectious agents occurs intracellularly, release of cytotoxic molecules into the extracellular milieu can damage body tissues."

In 1983, Clowes et al[62] reported on proteolytic activity in the plasma from patients with trauma or sepsis. A couple of years later, Moldawer et al[57] found that partially purified products of Staphylococcus albus-stimulated human blood monocytes increased skeletal protein degradation both in vivo and in vitro. However, neither the recombinant IL-1α, IL-1β nor TNF-α preparations had any impact on skeletal protein balance.

Goldberg et al[63] found an increase in net protein breakdown, induced by polypeptides released from porcine monocytes or serum from febrile cattles which had been injected with Pasteurella haemolytica or bovine rhinotracheitis. However, the macrophage product responsible for the protein breakdown was distinct from IL-1 and a number of other monokines.

Flores et al[64] investigated the effects on protein degradation of several doses of recombinant IL-1β and/or TNF-α. They found that muscle proteolysis was enhanced by TNF and synergistically enhanced by the addition of IL-1. More prolonged infusions of TNF and IL-1 increased the protein breakdown.

Nawabi et al[65] found that human recombinant TNF-α and/or IL-1α or IL-1β activate branched chain α-keto acid dehydrogenase (a rate-limiting enzyme for amino acid oxidation in skeletal muscle) and increase muscle protein breakdown.

Although conflicting reports have been published, most authors agree that a monocyte-derived factor is responsible for muscle protein breakdown. Generally, evidence from in vivo experiments indicates that IL-1 and TNF are involved in muscle protein catabolism, but in vitro experiments do not support this concept. It is possible that IL-1 and TNF require a cofactor or processing (i.e., cleavage), or they are intermediaries that induce another factor that acts on the muscle itself.

Cannon et al[66] observed increased immunohistochemical staining for IL-1β in muscle sections treated with anti-IL-1β IgG. Increased staining intensity for IL-1β was found up to 5 days after completing exercise. These findings are in accordance with the report in 1965 by Snell and Atkins,[67] who found endogenous pyrogen activity in normal rabbit muscle extracts using the rabbit pyrogen assay. The presence of IL-1 in skeletal muscles several days after the exercise suggests that IL-1 may be involved in prolonged skeletal muscle damage or protein breakdown, but it does not provide any information about the site of production. Although TNF-α was not detected in skeletal muscle, it cannot be excluded that small amounts (below detection limit) was present.

In a recent study, a prolonged eccentric exercise model was employed (Rohde et al, unpublished data). We showed that when the protein breakdown was limited by administration of branched chain amino acids during eccentric exercise, the IL-6 response was not diminished. This finding is compatible with the hypothesis that IL-6 precedes and causes the protein breakdown.

Apoptosis is a specific form of cell death that plays an important role in development and regulation of growth. Apoptosis, in comparance with necrosis, is characterized by an early degradation of the DNA into oligonucleosomal fragments. Apoptosis differs markedly from necrosis, the changes associated with cell death arising from injury. Apoptosis occurs without inducing a localized inflammatory response, whereas necrosis results in an inflammatory response.

The current view is that after eccentric exercise myofibers are mechanically damaged, and therefore an inflammatory and necrotic process occurs. In our opinion, there are no reasons to doubt that in relation to eccentric exercise, the initial muscle damage is due to a necrotic process. However, in a recent study Sandri et al[68] report that DNA damage is present in muscles of runner mice 2 days after spontaneously running for an entire night. In contrast DNA damage was absent in sedentary mice. These findings suggest that apoptosis is a late manifestation in skeletal muscle damage. Future studies will hopefully elucidate whether TNF plays a role in the apoptotic process in prolonged muscle damage.

There are several lines of evidence suggesting that cytokines, produced in response to exercise, may be involved in prolonged muscle damage and protein breakdown. However, in order to study the pathogenetic roles of cytokines, more sensitive methods such as polymerase chain reaction and in situ hybridization techniques are required.

CONCLUSION

Increased levels of inflammatory cytokines, primarily IL-6, have been found in response to exercise. The presence of multiple cytokines in urine following exercise shows that the expression of a broad spectrum of cytokines in response to exercise is possible.

A small increase in plasma IL-6 has been found after concentric exercise. However, high levels of cytokines are associated with exercise causing muscle damage. Neuroendocrine hormones studied so far are not responsible for the release of cytokines. The close association between the exercise-induced muscle damage and cytokine response give rise to two important questions: Do damaged skeletal muscle initiate the production of cytokines or do the cytokines induce muscle damage?

To answer these questions, we hereby put forth a model (Fig. 6.1) on muscle damage and cytokines. In relation to eccentric exercise, myofibers are mechanically damaged leading to necrosis and initiation of an inflammatory process. Hereby, the production of inflammatory cytokines are stimulated. The production of inflammatory cytokines further stimulate the development of an acute inflammatory response with accumulation in the muscle of neutrophils followed by macrophages. The cytokines stimulate infiltrating macrophages to produce prostaglandins, which are central in the sensation of delayed onset muscle pain. Furthermore, the inflammatory cytokines contribute either directly or indirectly to the prolonged muscle damage.

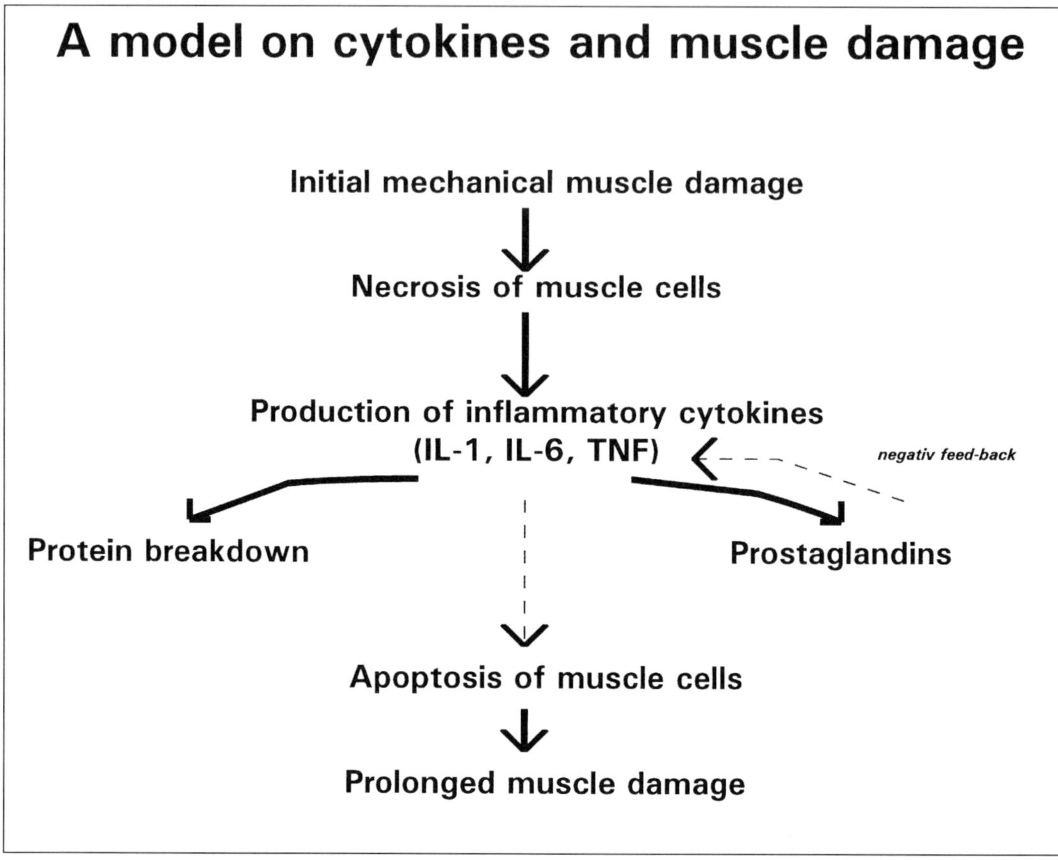

Fig. 6.1. A model is put forth on the possible relationship between cytokines and muscle damage: in relation to eccentric exercise, myofibers are mechanically damaged leading to initiation of an inflammatory process. The production of inflammatory cytokines stimulate the accumulation of neutrophils and macrophages in the muscle and contribute to the prolonged muscle damage.

References

1. Dinarello CA. Role of interleukin-1 in infectious diseases. Immunol Rev 1992; 127.
2. Dinarello CA, Wolff SM. The role of interleukin-1 in disease. N Engl J Med 1993; 328(2):106-113.
3. Seckinger P, Lowenthal JW, Williamson K et al. A urine inhibitor of interleukin 1 activity that blocks ligand binding. J Immunol 1987; 139(5):1546-1549.
4. Mazzei GJ, Seckinger PL, Dayer JM et al. Purification and characterization of a 26-kDa competitive inhibitor of interleukin 1. Eur J Immunol 1990; 20(3):683-689.

5. Hannum CH, Wilcox CJ, Arend WP et al. Interleukin-1 receptor antagonist activity of a human interleukin-1 inhibitor. Nature 1990; 343(6256):336-340.
6. Eisenberg SP, Evans RJ, Arend WP et al. Primary structure and functional expression from complementary DNA of a human interleukin-1 receptor antagonist. Nature 1990; 343(6256):341-346.
7. Dripps DJ, Brandhuber BJ, Thompson RC et al. Interleukin-1 (IL-1) receptor antagonist binds to the 80-kDa IL-1 receptor but does not initiate IL-1 signal transduction. J Biol Chem 1991; 266(16):10331-10336.
8. Granowitz EV, Clark BD, Mancilla J et al. Interleukin-1 receptor antagonist competitively inhibits the binding of interleukin-1 to the type II interleukin-1 receptor. J Biol Chem 1991; 266(22):14147-14150.
9. Van Snick J. Interleukin-6: an overview. Annu Rev Immunol 1990; 8.
10. Taga T, Kishimoto T. Cytokine receptors and signal transduction. FASEB J 1992; 6(15):3387-3396.
11. Vilcek J, Lee TH. Tumor necrosis factor. New insights into the molecular mechanisms of its multiple actions. J Biol Chem 1991; 266(12):7313-7316.
12. Beutler B, Cerami A. The biology of cachectin/TNF—a primary mediator of the host response. Annu Rev Immunol 1989; 7.
13. Smith CA, Davis T, Anderson D et al. A receptor for tumor necrosis factor defines an unusual family of cellular and viral proteins. Science 1990; 248(4958):1019-1023.
14. Loetscher H, Pan YC, Lahm HW et al. Molecular cloning and expression of the human 55 kd tumor necrosis factor receptor. Cell 1990; 61(2):351-359.
15. Engelmann H, Holtmann H, Brakebusch C et al. Antibodies to a soluble form of a tumor necrosis factor (TNF) receptor have TNF-like activity. J Biol Chem 1990; 265(24):14497-14504.
16. Tartaglia LA, Pennica D, Goeddel DV. Ligand passing: the 75-kDa tumor necrosis factor (TNF) receptor recruits TNF for signaling by the 55-kDa TNF receptor. J Biol Chem 1993; 268(25):18542-18548.
17. Tewari A, Buhles Jr WC, Starnes Jr HF. Preliminary report: effects of interleukin-1 on platelet counts. Lancet 1990; 336(8717):712-714.
18. Cannon JG, Kluger MJ. Endogenous pyrogen activity in human plasma after exercise. Science 1983; 220(4597):617-619.
19. Cannon JG, Evans WJ, Hughes VA et al. Physiological mechanisms contributing to increased interleukin-1 secretion. J Appl Physiol 1986; 61(5):1869-1874.
20. Evans WJ, Meredith CN, Cannon JG et al. Metabolic changes following eccentric exercise in trained and untrained men. J Appl Physiol 1986; 61(5):1864-1868.

21. Bagby GJ, Crouch LD, Shepherd RE. 4, Exercise and cytokines: Spontaneous and elicited response. In: Hoffman-Goetz L, ed. Exercise and immune function. New York: CRC Press, 1996:55-78.
22. Northoff H, Berg A. Immunologic mediators as parameters of the reaction to strenuous exercise. Int J Sports Med 1991; 12 (Suppl 1):S9-15.
23. Ullum H, Haahr PM, Diamant M et al. Bicycle exercise enhances plasma IL-6 but does not change IL-1α, IL-1β, IL-6, or TNF-α pre-mRNA in BMNC. J Appl Physiol 1994; 77(1):93-7.
24. Sprenger H, Jacobs C, Nain M et al. Enhanced release of cytokines, interleukin-2 receptors, and neopterin after long-distance running. Clin Immunol Immunopathol 1992; 63(2):188-95.
25. Cannon JG, Meydani SN, Fielding RA et al. Acute phase response in exercise. II. Associations between vitamin E, cytokines, and muscle proteolysis. Am J Physiol 1991; 260(6 Pt 2):R1235-40.
26. Rivier A, Pene J, Chanez P et al. Release of cytokines by blood monocytes during strenuous exercise. Int J Sports Med 1994; 15(4):192-8.
27. Smith JA, McKenzie SJ, Telford RD et al. Why does moderate exercise enhance, but intense training depress, immunity?. In: Husband, ed. Behavior and Immunity, 1992:155-68.
28. Ullum H, Palmø J, Halkjaer Kristensen J et al. The effect of acute exercise on lymphocyte subsets, natural killer cells, proliferative responses, and cytokines in HIV-seropositive persons. J Acquir Immune Defic Syndr 1994; 7(11):1122-1133.
29. Dufaux B, Order U. Plasma elastase-alpha 1-antitrypsin, neopterin, tumor necrosis factor, and soluble interleukin-2 receptor after prolonged exercise. Int J Sports Med 1989; 10:434-438.
30. Espersen GT, Elbaek A, Ernst E et al. Effect of physical exercise on cytokines and lymphocyte subpopulations in human peripheral blood. APMIS 1990; 98(5):395-400.
31. Viti A, Muscettola M, Paulesu L et al. The effects of exercise on plasma interferon levels. J Appl Physiol 1985; 59:426-429.
32. Bruunsgaard H, Galbo H, Halkjaer-Kristensen J et al. Exercise-induced increase in interleukin-6 is related to muscle damage. J Physiol Lond 1996; (in press).
33. Haahr PM, Pedersen BK, Fomsgaard A et al. Effect of physical exercise on in vitro production of interleukin 1, interleukin 6, tumor necrosis factor-alpha, interleukin 2 and interferon-gamma. Int J Sports Med 1991; 12(2):223-7.
34. Lewicki R, Tchorzewski H, Majewska E et al. Effect of Maximal Physical Exercise on T-Lymphocyte Subpopulations and on Interleukin 1 (IL-1) and Interleukin 2 (IL-2) Production in Vitro. Int J Sports Med 1988; 9:114-117.

35. Kvernmo H, Olsen JO, Osterud B. Changes in blood cell response following strenuous physical exercise. Eur J Appl Physiol 1992; 64(4):318-22.
36. Northoff H, Weinstock C, Berg A. The cytokine response to strenuous exercise. Int J Sports Med 1994; 15:S167-71.
37. Kasama TK, Kobayashi T, Fukushima M et al. Production of interleukin 1-like factor from human peripheral blood monocytes and polymorphonuclear leukocytes by superoxide anion: the role of interleukin 1 and reactive oxygen species in inflamed sites. Immunol Immunopathol 1989; 53:439-448.
38. Davies KJA, Packer L, Brooks GA. Free radicals and tissue produced by exercise. Biochem Biophys Res Commun 1982; 107:1198-1205.
39. Bagby GJ, Sawaya DE, Crouch LD et al. Prior exercise suppresses the plasma tumor necrosis factor response to bacterial lipopolysaccharide. J Appl Physiol 1994; 77(3):1542-7.
40. Camus G, Deby-Dupont G, Duhateau J et al. Are similar inflammatory factors involved in strenous exercise and sepsis? Intensive Care Med 1994; 20:602-610.
41. Bouchama A, Parhar RS, el Yazigi A et al. Endotoxemia and release of tumor necrosis factor and interleukin 1 alpha in acute heatstroke. J Appl Physiol 1991; 70(6):2640-2644.
42. DuBose DA, Basamania K, Maglione L et al. Role of bacterial endotoxins of intestinal origin in rat heat stress mortality. J Appl Physiol 1983; 54(1):31-36.
43. Brock Utne JG, Gaffin SL, Wells MT et al. Endotoxaemia in exhausted runners after a long-distance race. S Afr Med J 1988; 73(9):533-536.
44. Bosenberg AT, Brock Utne JG, Gaffin SL et al. Strenuous exercise causes systemic endotoxemia. J Appl Physiol 1988; 65(1):106-108.
45. Moore GE, Holbein ME, Knochel JP. Exercise-associated collapse in cyclists is unrelated to endotoxemia. Med Sci Sports Exerc 1995; 27(9):1238-1242.
46. Asmussen E. Positive and negative muscular work. Acta Physiol Scand 1953; 28:364-382.
47. Armstrong RB. Initial events in exercise-induced muscular injury. Med Sci Sports Exerc 1990; 22(4):429-435.
48. Friden J, Lieber RL. Structural and mechanical basis of exercise-induced muscle injury. Med Sci Sports Exerc 1992; 24(5):521-530.
49. Smith LL. Acute inflammation: the underlying mechanism in delayed onset muscle soreness? Med Sci Sports Exerc 1991; 23(5):542-551.
50. Pizza FX, Mitchell JB, Davis BH et al. Exercise-induced muscle damage: effect on circulating leukocyte and lymphocyte subsets. Med Sci Sports Exerc 1995; 27(3):363-370.

51. Francis KT, Hoobler T. Effects of aspirin on delayed muscle soreness. J Sports Med Phys Fitness 1987; 27(3):333-337.
52. Hikida RS, Staron RS, Hagerman FC et al. Muscle fiber necrosis associated with human marathon runners. J Neurol Sci 1983; 59(2):185-203.
53. Jones DA, Newham DJ, Round JM et al. Experimental human muscle damage: morphological changes in relation to other indices of damage. J Physiol Lond 1986; 375.
54. Jones DA, Newham DJ, Clarkson PM. Skeletal muscle stiffness and pain following eccentric exercise of the elbow flexors. Pain 1987; 30(2):233-242.
55. Dejana E, Bertocchi F, Bortolami MC et al. Interleukin 1 promotes tumor cell adhesion to cultured human endothelial cells. J Clin Invest 1988; 82:1466-1470.
56. Dinarello CA. Interleukin-1 and interleukin-1 antagonism. Blood 1991; 77(8):1627-1652.
57. Moldawer LL, Svaninger G, Gelin J et al. Interleukin 1 and tumor necrosis factor do not regulate protein balance in skeletal muscle. Am J Physiol 1987; 253(6 Pt 1):C766-C773.
58. de Vries HE, Hoogendoorn KH, van Dijk J et al. Eicosanoid production by rat cerebral endothelial cells: stimulation by lipopolysaccharide, interleukin-1 and interleukin-6. J Neuroimmunol 1995; 59(1-2):1-8.
59. Strassmann G, Patil Koota V, Finkelman F et al. Evidence for the involvement of interleukin 10 in the differential deactivation of murine peritoneal macrophages by prostaglandin E2. J Exp Med 1994; 180(6):2365-2370.
60. Ryan GB, Majno G. Acute inflammation. Am J Pathol 1977; 86:185-264.
61. Smith JA. Neutrophils, host defense, and inflammation: a double-edged sword. J Leukoc Biol 1994; 56(6):672-686.
62. Clowes GH, George BC, Villeee BC et al. Muscle proteolysis induced by a circulating peptide in patients with sepsis or trauma. N Engl J Med 1983; 308:545-552.
63. Goldberg AL, Kettelhut IC, Furuno K et al. Activation of protein breakdown and prostaglandin E2 production in rat skeletal muscle in fever is signaled by a macrophage product distinct from interleukin 1 or other known monokines. J Clin Invest 1988; 81(5):1378-1383.
64. Flores EA, Bistrian BR, Pomposelli JJ et al. Infusion of tumor necrosis factor/cachectin promotes muscle metabolism in the rat. A synergistic effect with interleukin 1. J Clin Invest 1989; 83(5):1614-1622.
65. Nawabi MD, Block KP, Chakrabarti MC et al. Administration of endotoxin, tumor necrosis factor, or interleukin 1 to rats activates

skeletal muscle branched-chain alpha-keto acid dehydrogenase. J Clin Invest 1990; 85:256-263.
66. Cannon JG, Fielding RA, Fiatarone MA et al. Increased interleukin 1 beta in human skeletal muscle after exercise. Am J Physiol 1989; 257(2 Pt 2):R451-455.
67. Snell ES, Atkins E. The presence of endogenous pyrogen in normal rabbit tissue. J Exp Med 1965; 121:1019-1038.
68. Sandri M, Carraro U, Podhorska-Okolov M et al. Apoptosis, DNA damage and ubiquitin expression in normal and mdx muscle fibers after exercise. FEBS Lett 1995; 373:291-295.

CHAPTER 7

Chronic Exercise and the Immune System

Bente Klarlund Pedersen

In contrast to a large number of studies on the immune response to acute exercise, much less is known concerning the effect of physical conditioning or training on immune function.

This is largely due to the difficulties in separating fitness effects from actual physical exercise. Thus, the changes induced by intense physical exercise may last at least 24 hours, and even moderate acute exercise induces significant immune changes for several hours. As it is not easy to persuade athletes to abstain from their normal training program even for just 1 day, it may be difficult to obtain results on true "resting levels." The influence of chronic exercise has been studied in both animal and human models, the latter including both longitudinal as well as cross-sectional studies.

CROSS-SECTIONAL HUMAN STUDIES

A good indicator of chronic exercise as a lifestyle factor is to compare resting levels of the immune system in untrained controls and in athletes who have been competing for several years. Two studies have been conducted on competitive male cyclists. In order to eliminate the effects of acute exercise in these studies, none of the subjects were allowed to exercise 20 hours prior to blood sampling. They all belonged to the elite Danish cycling group, and they had been active in sports for a median of 4 years and had trained a medium of 20,000 km per year. In the first study, the natural killer (NK) activity was measured in 27 highly trained cyclists and in 15 age- and sex-matched untrained controls. Median NK cell activity was 38.1% in the trained group compared to 30.3% in the untrained group ($p = 0.008$), and median %CD16$^+$ NK cells was 17% in the trained group versus 11% in the untrained group ($p = 0.007$).[1] An additional study[2] examined the cellular immune system in 29 cyclists and 15 controls, measures were taken under resting conditions during a period of low intensity training (winter). Fifteen cyclists and 10 controls were re-examined during a period of high intensity training (summer). The NK cell activity was significantly elevated in the trained group, both during the period of low intensity training (39.2% vs. 30.9%) and during the period of high intensity training (55.2% vs. 33.6%) (Fig. 7.1a).[2] During low intensity training, we found that the increased NK cell activity in trained subjects was due to an increased percentage of NK cells in these subjects. However, during high intensity training we found increased NK cell function in the trained subjects, despite a comparable number of circulating NK cells in trained subjects and controls (Fig. 7.1b). The mechanisms of this enhanced activity might be secondary to differences in NK cell activation. The results suggested that the NK cells were activated in trained subjects during high intensity training and that this may lead to an adjustment of the number of CD16$^+$ cells in circulation by some unknown mechanism. In these studies,[1,2] other lymphocyte subpopulations and the lymphocyte proliferative response did not differ among trained and untrained subjects.

Another study by Nieman et al[3] supported the finding that athletes have increased NK cell activity. The study[3] included 22 marathon runners who had completed at least seven marathons and had been training for marathon race events for at least 4 years. They were compared with a group of 18 sedentary controls. Despite a large difference between groups with regard to VO_2max, percent body fat and physical activity, only the NK cell activity among the immune system variables measured emerged as being significantly different between the groups (higher among the marathoners). Concentrations of leukocytes and lymphocyte subsets as well as mitogen-stimulated proliferative responses did not differ significantly between the groups.

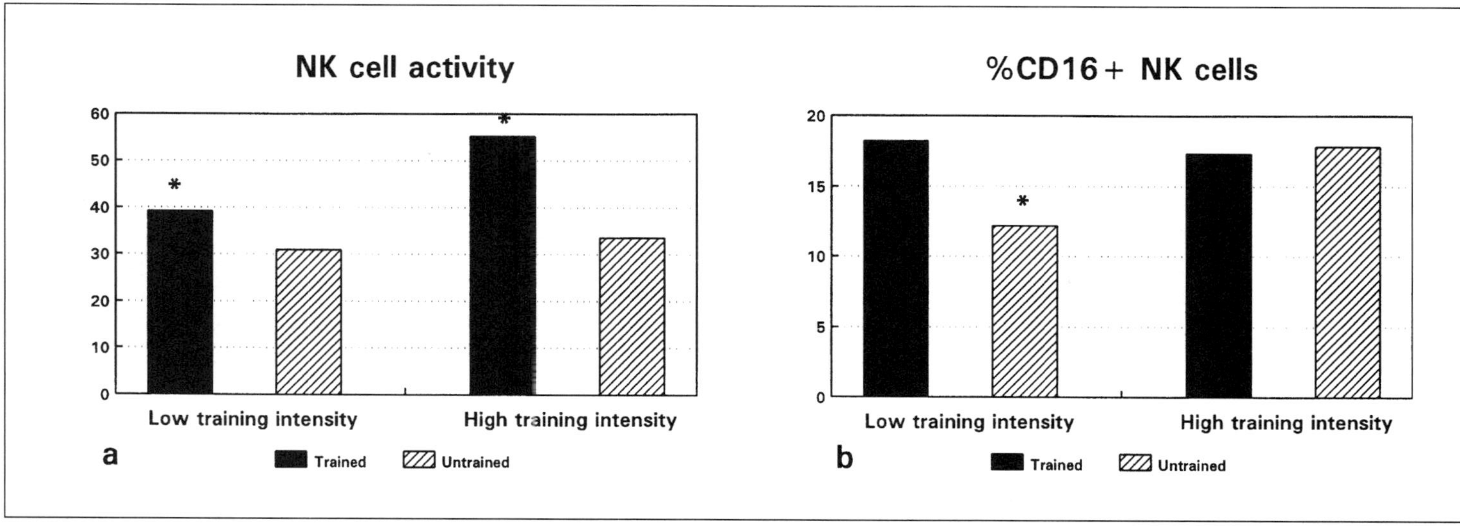

Fig. 7.1. Natural killer (NK) cell activity and %CD16+ NK cells of blood mononuclear cells (BMNC) isolated from trained and untrained individuals during high (summer) and low (winter) training intensities. VO_2max was median 72.0 ml/kg/minutes in trained and median 54.7 ml/kg/minutes in untrained. Trained subjects were male racing elite cyclists. * denotes significant difference among groups. Results are adapted from Tvede et al.[2]

Nieman et al[4] compared resting levels of several immune parameters in a group of 12 highly conditioned and 30 sedentary elderly women (67-85 years-old). The NK cell activity and phytohemagglutinin (PHA) stimulated proliferative responses were significantly elevated in the highly conditioned group compared with the inactive group.

In contrast to these studies, Brahmi et al[5] found no differences in NK cell activity when he compared 5 trained males and 10 untrained females and males. Furthermore, Nieman et al[6] compared 18 young male endurance athletes (10 runners and 8 cyclists) with 11 nonathletic male adults and found no difference regarding NK cell activity. For all subjects combined there was no correlation between immune function and VO_2max.

The lymphocyte proliferative response has been described to be either decreased,[7] elevated[4,8] or in most studies unchanged[1-3,6,9] when comparing athletes and nonathletes. The neutrophil function has been described to be either suppressed[10-12] or not significantly different[13,14] between trained and untrained groups. Baj et al[8] and Hack et al[15] found that the neutrophil function was unchanged in athletes during a low training period, but decreased during periods of high intensity training. Thus, there is a tendency towards decreased neutrophil function in athletes during periods of high intensity training.

LONGITUDINAL HUMAN STUDIES

The effect of chronic exercise has been studied in longitudinal designs. This is advantageous as the studies use randomization, thus in principle excluding confounding factors. The disadvantage is that the majority of studies investigate the effect on the immune system of at most 16 weeks of training, whereas the cross-sectional studies reflect many years of training. All studies, however, show significant effects on VO_2max as a result of training.

Nieman et al[4] found no influence on NK cell activity or any other immune parameters, when 30 elderly women were randomized into a 12 week walking program, whereas Crist et al[16] found that treadmill exercise for 16 weeks enhanced the NK cell activity in elderly women. In another study, Nieman et al[17] found that

15 weeks of walking enhanced the NK cell activity in moderately obese, previously inactive women. When 18 patients with rheumatoid arthritis were allocated to an 8 week cycling program, it was found that chronic exercise had no effect on the NK cell activity, lymphocyte proliferative responses, concentrations or proportions of lymphocyte subpopulation or cytokine production.[18] Furthermore, exercise had no influence on erythrocyte sedimentation rate, C reactive protein or number of swollen and tender joints. However, using a visual analog scale it was shown that the patients who had performed the exercise program had less pain, less morning stiffness and were less fatigued. It is interesting that the studies with the longest followup period demonstrate a positive effect of chronic training on NK activity.

REPEATED BOUTS OF EXERCISE

The effects of chronic exercise or repeated exercise on the immune response to one bout of acute exercise has been investigated in a few studies. Ndon[19] showed that the leukocyte response to an acute bout of exercise in trained athletes was not altered during 28 days of chronic intense training. Repeated bouts of acute submaximal exercise on days 1, 3 and 5 resulted in similar increases in the percentage of NK cells,[20] whereas six repeated bouts of maximal intense exercise (rowing) over 2 days provoked higher immune responses during the repetitive bouts of exercise. Interestingly, resting levels of the lymphocyte count and NK cell activity were elevated the day after the exercise was completed.[21]

ANIMAL STUDIES

MacNeil and Hoffman-Goetz[22] investigated the influence of 9 weeks of chronic exercise on natural cytotoxicity in male C3H mice. Both in vivo cytotoxicity (pulmonary vasculature) and in vitro cytotoxicity (spleen) were determined for voluntary (wheel running) and forced (treadmill running, 15 mi/minute, 30 minutes/day) training. A sedentary control group and a treadmill control group (5 m/minutes, 5 minutes/day) were included. Forced and voluntary chronic exercise enhanced in vivo as well as in vitro cytotoxic activity in comparison with both the control groups.

Several studies from the same group, using training protocols of varying length and intensity and different animal species, support the findings showing increased resting levels of natural cytotoxicity after voluntary exercise.[23-26]

Lin et al[27] examined the effect of chronic exercise training in rats, who were trained on a drum exerciser at the intensity of 60-70% of VO_2max for 30 minutes and then extended up to 60 minutes per day, 5 days per week. The rats were at rest 3 days before sacrifice, and it was found that the interleukin (IL)-2 production was suppressed in the training group.

IMMUNE FUNCTION AND DIETARY FACTORS IN ATHLETES

Cross-sectional studies in humans including 27,[1] 29,[2] 12[4] and 22[3] athletes show that the NK cell activity is increased in trained versus untrained subjects; however, two studies including 5[5] and 18[6] athletes did not confirm this. The longitudinal studies have shown variable influence of training on the immune system[4,16,17,28] in humans. Regarding lymphocyte proliferation, there are no consistent findings, whereas there is a tendency towards suppressed neutrophil function in periods of intense training.[8,15] Is it possible that the divergent findings on chronic exercise/training and natural immunity, reflect that life style factors related with exercise training, such as the diet, influence the immune system.

Nieman et al[3] found that percent body fat was negatively correlated with the NK cell activity. Similar findings were reported by the same group in a study including 42 elderly females.[4] It has recently been concluded that although research data on humans are limited, obesity does appear to be associated with impaired immune function.[29] Although the data on NK cell activity and obesity is limited, it is possible that the increased level of NK cell activity in athletes is not directly related to training, but dependent on other lifestyle factors, such as diet.

The fatty acid composition of the diet can alter the fatty acid composition of immunocompetent cells. Changes in the fatty acid profiles of the plasma membranes may also alter the membrane fluidity and the eicosanoids produced, which in turn may alter the activity of the immune cells.[30] Interestingly, it was found that the NK cell activity increased in young men after 12 weeks on a low-fat diet in which both saturated and nonsaturated fatty acid content in the diet was lowered.[31] In another study, however, the immune system, including the NK cell activity, was not influenced by the two different diets consisting of either 6 weeks of a lacto-ovo vegetarian diet or 6 weeks of a mixed Western diet.[32] The lack of influence on the immune system in the latter study may be due the short study period, as it takes 12 weeks to alter the lipid composition of the lymphocyte membranes.

There have only been few studies in humans investigating the influence of fat-type on immune function. A negative correlation between linoleic acid in blood mononuclear cells and NK cell activity was found in healthy controls,[33] and this finding was confirmed in a study examining elderly men.[34] Thus, although several studies tend to show that immune function is enhanced by low-fat diet,[31,35-38] the conclusion so far is less clear for the type of dietary fat.

CONCLUSION

NK cell activity is increased in athletes versus nonathletes, however, in randomized, longitudinal studies chronic training has not shown a consistent effect on NK cell activity. This may be explained by the following: in order to become a successful athlete, good health is an absolute necessity. Thus, the level of natural immunity may select who will be an athlete and who will not, and the cross-sectional studies may in theory simply reflect this selection. However, whereas the longitudinal training studies in humans fail to show consistent effects on natural immunity, most animal studies have shown that chronic exercise enhances resting levels of natural cytotoxic activity. The latter indicates a true relationship, not just an association, between NK cell activity and chronic exercise. Thus, a high level of resting natural immunity exists in trained individuals. How do we then explain the fact that elite athletes as a group are more prone to upper respiratory tract infections than their sedentary counterparts? The most likely explanation is that the increased susceptibility to infections is due to postexercise suppression of NK and B cell functions. During this postexercise temporary immunosuppression[39] there is an "open window" of opportunity for pathogens.[40] In a recent review on the regulation of neutrophil function during exercise, Pyne[11] suggests that repetitive high-intensity training sessions by elite athletes may leave a significant proportion of their circulating neutrophils in a chronically refractory state. This may also explain the observation that elite athletes, as a group, are more susceptible to infections.[41]

References

1. Pedersen BK, Tvede N, Christensen LD et al. Natural killer cell activity in peripheral blood of highly trained and untrained persons. Int J Sports Med 1989; 10(2):129-131.
2. Tvede N, Steensberg J, Baslund B et al. Cellular immunity in highly trained elite racing cyclists during periods of training with high and low intensity. Scand J Med Sci Sports 1991; 1:163-6.
3. Nieman DC, Buckley KS, Henson DA et al. Immune function in marathon runners versus sedentary controls. Med Sci Sports Exerc 1995; 27(7):986-992.
4. Nieman DC, Henson DA, Gusewitch G et al. Physical activity and immune function in elderly women. Med Sci Sports Exerc 1993; 25(7):823-831.
5. Brahmi Z, Thomas JE, Park M et al. The effect of acute exercise on natural killer-cell activity of trained and sedentary human subjects. J Clin Immunol 1985; 5(5):321-328.
6. Nieman DC, Brendle D, Henson DA et al. Immune function in athletes versus nonathletes. Int J Sports Med 1995; 16(5):329-33.
7. Papa S, Vitale M, Mazzotti G et al. Impaired lymphocyte stimulation induced by longterm training. Immunol Lett 1989; 22:29-33.
8. Baj Z, Kantorski J, Majewska E et al. Immunological status of competitive cyclists before and after the training season. Int J Sports Med 1994; 15(6):319-24.
9. Oshida Y, Yamanouchi K, Hayamizu S et al. Effect of acute physical exercise on lymphocyte subpopulations in trained and untrained subjects. Int J Sports Med 1988; 9(2):137-140.
10. Lewicki R, Tchorzewski H, Majewska E et al. Effect of Maximal Physical Exercise on T-Lymphocyte Subpopulations and on Interleukin 1 (IL-1) and Interleukin 2 (IL-2) Production in Vitro. Int J Sports Med 1988; 9:114-117.
11. Pyne DB. Regulation of neutrophil function during exercise. Sports Med 1994; 17(4):245-58.
12. Ahlborg B. Leukocytes in blood during prolonged physical exercise. Forsvarsmedicin 1967; 3:36-48.

13. Hack V, Strobel G, Rau JP et al. The effect of maximal exercise on the activity of neutrophil granulocytes in highly trained athletes in a moderate training period. Eur J Appl Physiol 1992; 65(6):520-4.
14. Green RL, Kaplan SS, Rabin BS et al. Immune function in marathon runners. Ann Allergy 1981; 47(2):73-75.
15. Hack V, Strobel G, Weiss M et al. PMN cell counts and phagocytic activity of highly trained athletes depend on training period. J Appl Physiol 1994; 77(4):1731-5.
16. Crist DM, Mackinnon LT, Thompson RF et al. Physical Exercise Increases Natural Cellular-Mediated Tumor Cytotoxity in Elderly Women. Gerontology 1989; 35:66-71.
17. Nieman DC, Nehlsen Cannarella SL, Markoff PA et al. The effects of moderate exercise training on natural killer cells and acute upper respiratory tract infections. Int J Sports Med 1990; 11(6):467-473.
18. Baslund B, Lyngberg K, Andersen V et al. Effect of 8 wk of bicycle training on the immune system of patients with rheumatoid arthritis. J Appl Physiol 1993; 75(4):1691-5.
19. Ndon JA, Snyder AC, Foster C et al. Effects of chronic intense exercise training on the leukocyte response to acute exercise. Int J Sports Med 1992; 13(2):176-82.
20. Hoffman-Goetz L, Simpson JR, Cipp N et al. Lymphocyte subset responses to repeated submaximal exercise in men. J Appl Physiol 1990; 68(3):1069-1074.
21. Nielsen HB, Secher N, Perdersen BK. Lymphocytes and NK cell activity during repeated bouts of maximal exercise. Am J Physiol 1996; 271:R222-R227.
22. MacNeil B, Hoffman-Goetz L. Chronic exercise enhances in vivo and in vitro cytotoxic mechanisms of natural immunity in mice. J Appl Physiol 1993; 74(1):388-95.
23. Hoffman-Goetz L, Arumugam Y, Sweeny L. Lymphokine activated killer cell activity following voluntary physical activity in mice. J Sports Med Phys Fit 1994; 34:83-90.
24. Hoffman-Goetz L, MacNeil B, Arumugam Y et al. Differential effects of exercise and housing condition on murine natural killer cell activity and tumor growth. Int J Sports Med 1992; 13(2):167-71.
25. MacNeil B, Hoffman-Goetz L. Effect of exercise on natural cytotoxicity and pulmonary tumor metastases in mice. Med Sci Sports Exerc 1993; 25(8):922-8.
26. MacNeil B, Hoffman-Goetz L. Exercise training and tumor metastasis in mice: influence of time of exercise onset. Anticancer Res 1993; 13(6A):2085-8.
27. Lin YS, Jan MS, Chen HI. The effect of chronic and acute exercise on immunity in rats. Int J Sports Med 1993; 14(2):86-92.

28. Barnes CA, Forster MJ, Fleshner M et al. Exercise does not modify spatial memory, brain autoimmunity, or antibody response in aged F-344 rats. Neurobiol Aging 1991; 12(1):47-53.
29. Stallone DD. The influence of obesity and its treatment on the immune system. Nutr Rev 1994; 52(2 Pt 1):37-50.
30. Kelley DS, Daudu PA. Fat intake and immune response. Prog Food Nutr Sci 1993; 17(1):41-63.
31. Barone J, Herbert JR, Reddy MM. Dietary fat and natural-killer-cell activity. Am J Clin Nutr 1989; 50:861-867.
32. Richter EA, Kiens B, Raben A et al. Immune parameters in male atheletes after a lacto-ovo vegetarian diet and a mixed Western diet. Med Sci Sports Exerc 1991; 23(5):517-21.
33. Oxholm P, Pedersen BK, Horrobin DF. Natural killer cell functions are related to the cell membrane composition of essential fatty acids: differences in healthy persons and patients with primary Sjogren's syndrome. Clin Exp Rheumatol 1992; 10(3):229-234.
34. Rasmussen LB, Kiens B, Pedersen BK et al. Effect of diet and plasma fatty acid composition on immune status in elderly men. Am J Clin Nutr 1994; 59(3):572-577.
35. McHugh MI, Wilkinson R, Elliot RW et al. Immunosupression with polyunsaturated fatty acids in renal transplantation. Transplantation 1977; 24:263-267.
36. Erickson KL, McNiell CJ, Gershwin ME et al. Influence of dietary fat concentration and saturation on immune ontogeny in mice. J Nutr 1980; 110:1555-1572.
37. Locniskar M, Nauss KM, Newberne PM. The effect of quality and quantity of dietary fat on the immune system. J Nutr 1983; 113:951-961.
38. Kelly DS, Branch LB, Iacono JM. Nutritional modulation of human immune status. Nutr Res 1989; 9:956-975.
39. Pedersen BK, Ullum H. NK cell response to physical activity: possible mechanisms of action. Med Sci Sports Exerc 1994; 26:(2):140-6.
40. Brines R, Hoffman-Goetz L, Pedersen BK. Can you exercise to make your immune system fitter? Immunol Today 1996; 17(6):252-254.
41. Nieman DC. 8, Prolonged aerobic exercise, immune response, and risk of infection. In: Hoffman-Goetz L, ed. Exercise and Immune Function. New York: CRC Press, 1996:143-162.

CHAPTER 8

Exercise in Patients with HIV Infection

Bente Klarlund Pedersen and Henrik Ullum

Given the fact that both acute and chronic exercise modulates the immune system, it is obviously important to determine how exercise influences the immune system in immunosuppressed patients such as in patients infected with the human immunodeficiency virus (HIV). The primary immunologic defect in individuals infected with HIV is a depletion of the $CD4^+$ T cell subset.[1,2] However, conjoint effects have been reported on the function of other lymphocyte subpopulations, including the natural killer (NK) cells and lymphokine activated killer (LAK) cells.[3]

ACUTE EXERCISE

In healthy subjects, exercise-induced alterations in the immune system include changes in blood mononuclear cells (BMNC), proliferative responses as well as NK and LAK cell functions.[4] A study on acute exercise[5] was designed to determine to what extent HIV-infected individuals were able to mobilize immunocompetent cells to the blood in response to physical exercise. The study included eight asymptomatic men infected with HIV and eight HIV-seronegative controls, who cycled for 1 hour at 75% of VO_2max. The percentages of $CD4^+$, $CD4^+45RA^+$, $CD4^+45RO^+$ cells did not change in response to exercise, whereas the concentration of $CD4^+$ cells increased two-fold during exercise (Fig. 8.1).

Exercise Immunology, edited by Bente Klarlund Pedersen. © 1997 R.G. Landes Company.

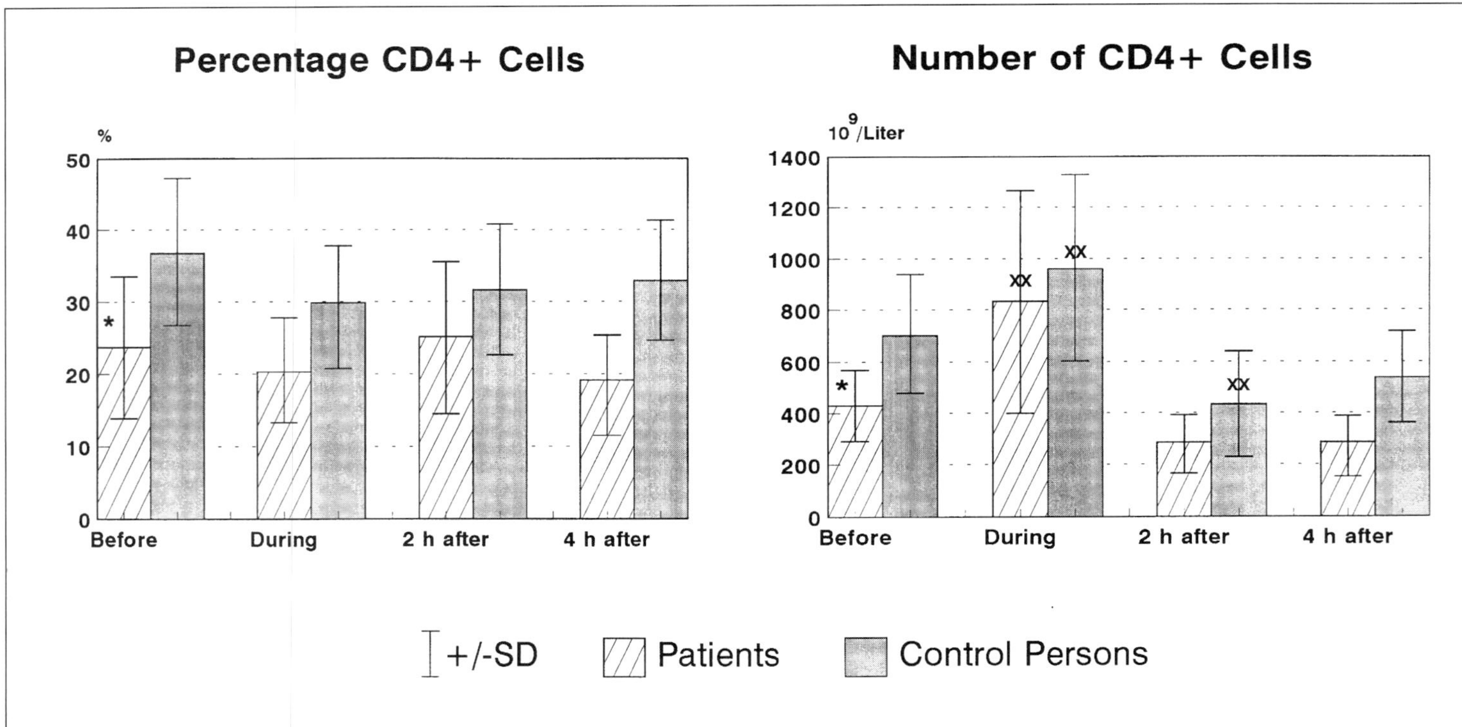

Fig. 8.1. The effect of bicycle exercise 75% of VO_2max, 1 hour, on percentage and absolute numbers of $CD4^+$ cells in human immunodeficiency syndrome (HIV)-seropositive individuals ($n = 8$) and controls ($n = 8$). Means and SD are shown. *denotes significant difference between HIV-seropositive and control group ($p < 0.05$); xx denotes significant differences from preexercise values ($p < 0.01$). Reprinted with permission from Ullum H et al, J Acquir Immune Defic Syndr 1994; 7(11):1122-1133.

The level of $CD4^+$ cells in the circulation has prognostic value for predicting the development of acquired immunodeficiency syndrome (AIDS)[6-8] in HIV-infected patients and for predicting mortality resulting from complications of HIV infection in AIDS.[9,10] However, increases in the concentration of $CD4^+$ cells (the CD4 count) and CD4 percentage in response to treatment may not always reflect a better prognosis.[11,12]

It has been debated which of the immunological markers to use: the absolute number or the percentage of $CD4^+$ cells. Taylor et al[13] showed that the percentage of $CD4^+$ lymphocytes had slightly greater prognostic significance and showed slightly less variability on repeated measurement. The finding that the CD4 count, but not the percentage of $CD4^+$ cells changed in response to acute exercise, offers one explanation of the variability in the absolute numbers of $CD4^+$ cells. Furthermore, it also strengthens the idea that the percentage of $CD4^+$ cells is preferable to the number of $CD4^+$ cells in monitoring patients seropositive for HIV.

Interestingly, HIV-seropositive subjects were shown to possess an impaired ability to mobilize neutrophils (Fig. 8.2) and cells mediating NK cell activity (Fig. 8.3). Furthermore, only control persons showed increased LAK cell activity in the blood in response to exercise, whereas HIV-seropositive subjects did not.[5] Because exercise is accepted as a model of physical stress, the study on acute exercise suggests that HIV-seropositive subjects, although only moderately immunosuppressed, possess an impaired ability to generate unspecific immunity towards microbial agents in response to various physical stimuli.

The mechanisms behind the defective recruitment of cells to the blood are not fully understood, but may include: (1) an impaired stress hormone response (e.g., the increase in catecholamines and growth hormone during physical exercise may be lower in HIV-seropositive subjects); (2) low expression of β-receptors on the surface of NK cells; or (3) alternatively, HIV-seropositive persons may simply have a smaller reservoir of cells available for recruitment.[14]

CHRONIC EXERCISE

Chronic exercise or training have been described in most studies to have no effect on lymphocyte proliferation in healthy HIV-

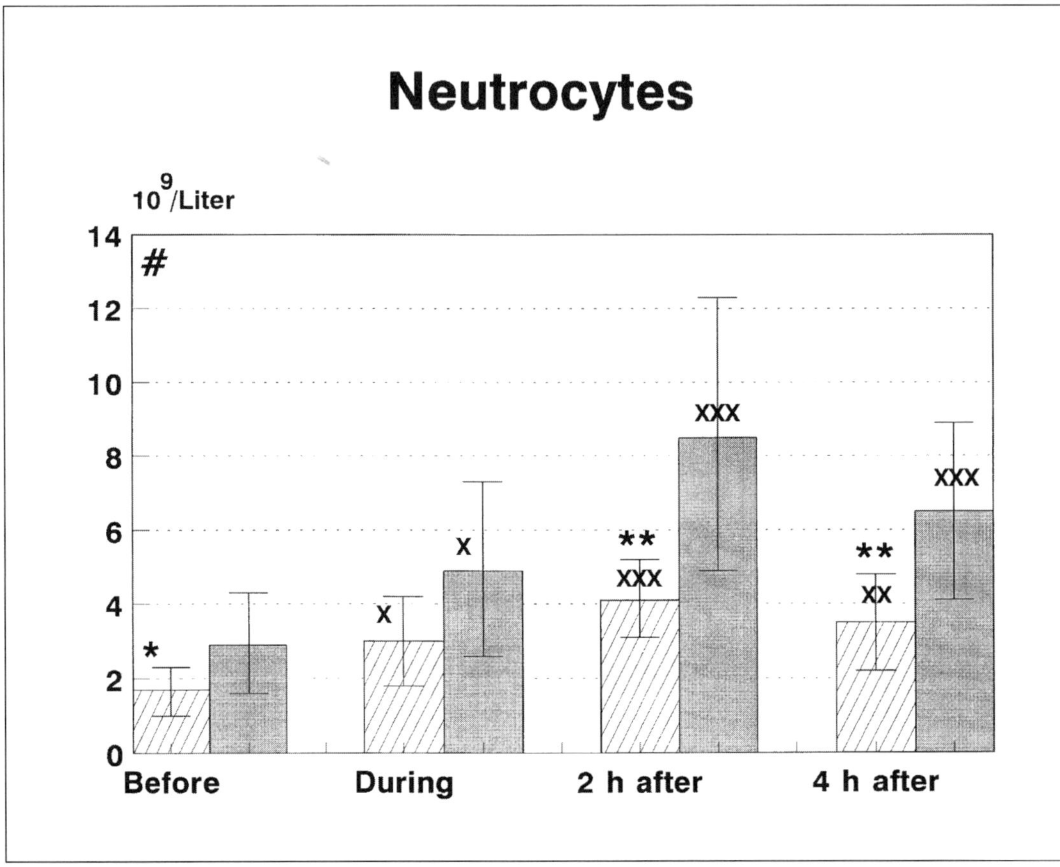

*Fig. 8.2. The effect of bicycle exercise 75% of VO_2max 1 hour on concentrations of neutrophils in human immunodeficiency syndrome (HIV)- seropositive individuals ($n = 8$) and controls ($n = 8$). Means and SD are shown, # denotes significant interference between time and HIV-seropositive status by three-way factorial analysis. * denotes significant difference between HIV-seropositive and control group ($p < 0.05$) (**$p < 0.01$), x denotes significant difference between HIV-seropositive and control group ($p < 0.05$) (xx; $p < 0.01$, xxx; $p < 0.001$). Reprinted with permission from Ullum H et al, J Acquir Immune Defic Syndr 1994; 7(11):1122-1133.*

seronegative individuals.[15-19] One study showed that chronic exercise enhanced resting levels of the CD4 count,[20] although most studies found no effect on concentrations or percentages of $CD4^+$ cells in HIV-seronegative subjects.[15-18,21-24] However, trained HIV-seronegative athletes have been reported to have enhanced resting levels of NK cell function compared to untrained subjects.[4,22,24,25]

There are only few controlled studies on the effect of chronic exercise on the immune system in HIV-seropositive subjects. Rigsby et al[26] performed a controlled, randomized study, including 19

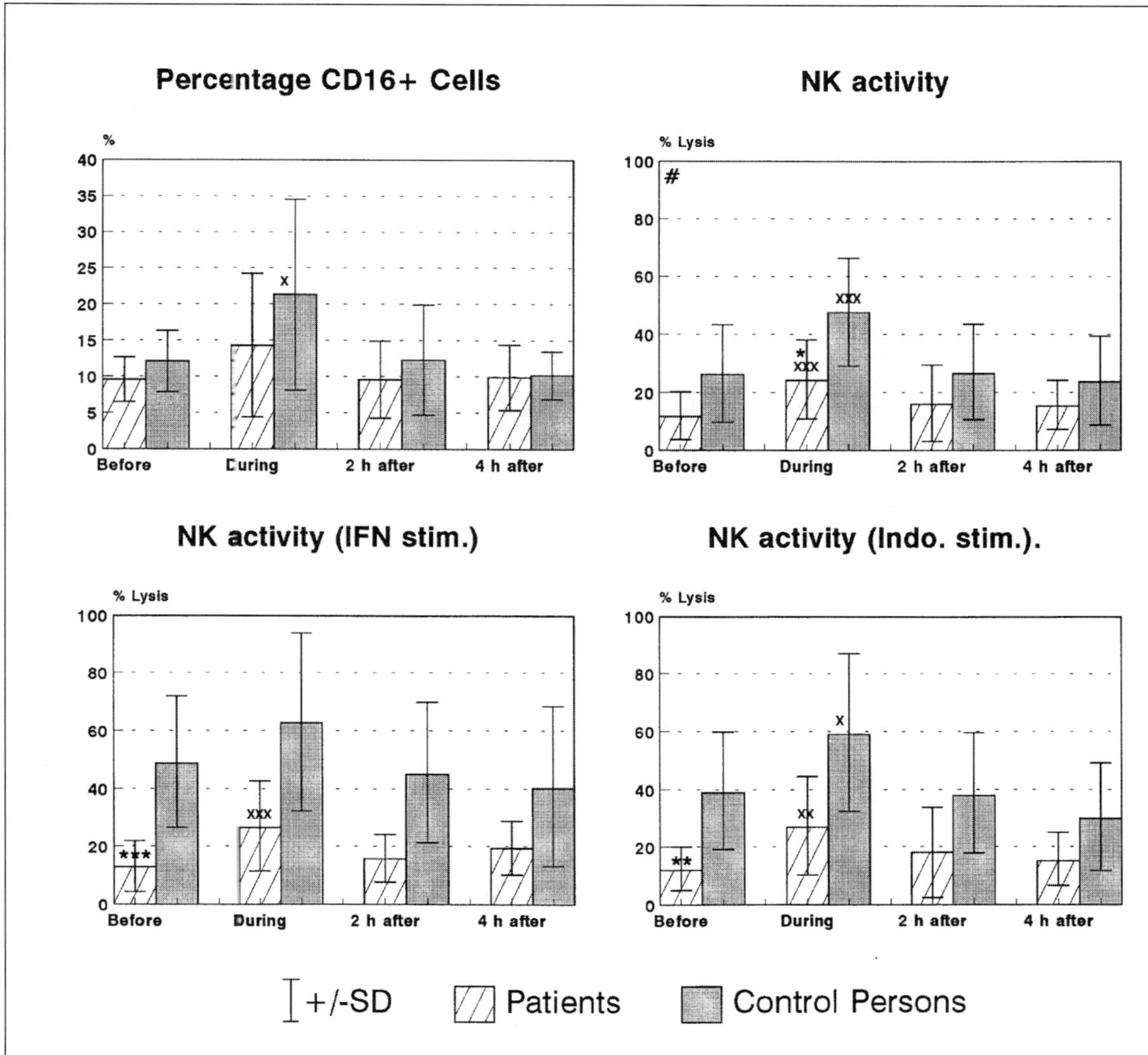

*Fig. 8.3. The effect of bicycle exercise 75% of VO_2max, 1 hour, on %$CD16^+$ natural killer (NK) cells, unstimulated, interferon-α-stimulated (IFN-stim) and indomethacin-stimulated (indo-stim) NK cell activity in HIV-seropositive (n = 8) and HIV-seronegative individuals (n = 8). Means and SD are shown, # denotes significant difference interference between time and HIV-seropositive status by three-way factorial analysis. * denotes significant difference between HIV-seropositive and control group ($p < 0.05$) (**$p < 0.01$, ***$p < 0.001$), x denotes significant differences from preexercise values ($p < 0.05$) (xx; $p < 0.01$, xxx; $p < 0.001$). Reprinted with permission from Ullum H et al, J Acquir Immune Defic Syndr 1994; 7(11): 1122-1133.*

HIV-seropositive subjects—groups II, III and IV according to Center for Disease Control (CDC)—who performed bicycle exercise training for 12 weeks. Eighteen HIV-seropositive individuals, who did not exercise, were included as controls. Immune monitoring included flow cytometry analysis of lymphocyte subpopulations. Although training induced significant increases in neuromuscular strength and cardiorespiratory fitness, there was no significant effects on the CD4 count or other lymphocyte subpopulations.

A similar randomized, controlled training study was performed by LaPerriere et al.[27] The study included 10 HIV-seropositive subjects who performed bicycle exercise training for 45 minutes three times a week for 10 weeks. The study also included HIV-seropositive control subjects who did not train. The CD4 count, the CD56 count and the NK cell activity measured per $CD56^+$ cell in whole blood were reported not to change as a result of training. However, a later review article by LaPerriere et al[28] reported increases in the CD4 count and in the number of $CD4^+CD45RA^+$ cells.[27] Birk et al[29] included five HIV-seropositive subjects in a 1 year training study, and MacArthur et al[30] studied six HIV-seropositive subjects, CDC stage IV, who performed 24 weeks of training. Training had no effect on the CD4 count in either of the studies.[29,30]

One study, unfortunately, does not report the number of dropouts.[27] However, other studies reported 1 of 5 (29%),[29] 4 of 23 (17%)[26] and 19 of 25 (76%)[30] dropouts. Clinical deterioration in some patients is probably a major cause of the high dropout rates reported in training studies including seropositive patients. Thus, although Rigsby et al[26] did not find differences between the training group and the control group regarding the number of subjects who dropped out or died, it cannot be excluded that HIV-seropositive subjects dropped out because exercise training worsened their disease. These dropouts therefore constitute a clinically very important group. If training induces an immunological and clinical deterioration in some patients, who then dropped out of the training program, this would be a major source of error.

Some of the studies have shown an insignificant increase in CD4 count in patients that train. Based on these results it has been concluded that training increases the CD4 count in HIV-seropositive patients.[28] This is a very important conclusion since it could lead to the acceptance of physical training as a treatment of HIV infection. However, no study has to our knowledge been able to show any significant effect of training on the CD4 count in HIV infected patients. If patients with declining CD4 counts drop out of the exercise regimen due to declining health this could lead to a false impression of an increasing CD4 count caused by physical training.

Recently, the ability to measure HIV-RNA in plasma has contributed to our understanding of the pathogenesis of the HIV infection. Recent data demonstrate that a continuous high replication of HIV leads to an exhaustion of the vast proliferative capacity of the immune system; in other words, the destruction of the $CD4^+$ T cells eventually exceed their replenishment.[31,32] The use of both CD4 counts and plasma HIV-RNA measurements in the monitoring of HIV infected patients has added greatly to the prognostic value of the isolated use of the CD4 count for predicting progression of the HIV infection. Furthermore, the concomitant measurement of β_2-microglobulin is a useful prognostic marker for predicting disease progression. Thus, in order to accept exercise as a treatment of HIV infection, exercise must be shown not only to increase CD4 counts but also to reduce the viral load and the immunological activation as expressed by plasma HIV-RNA and serum β_2-microglobulin. Furthermore, since HIV infection is known to inhibit the function of the cellular immune response, a true positive clinical effect of any treatment of HIV infection would also lead to increases in the functional capacity of the cellular immune system.

However, there are a lack of studies on the effect of training on viral load as measured by plasma HIV-RNA and β_2-microglobulin. Furthermore, there are no data showing a beneficial effect of training on resting levels of lymphocyte proliferation and cytotoxic functions in HIV-seropositive individuals.

Thus, any encouragement for HIV-seropositive patients to perform physical exercise relies on the positive effect on muscle strength and oxygen uptake and the psychological relief accomplished in the patients that are able to participate in a training program.

CONCLUSION

HIV-seropositive patients have an impaired ability to mobilize neutrophils, NK and LAK cells to the blood in response to acute exercise. However, it is not known if this finding can be extended to other stressors, that is if the immune reactions to stress in general is impaired. There are no consistent findings regarding an effect of chronic training on resting levels of the immune system in HIV-seropositive patients. Therefore, the available amount of data does not allow us to draw any conclusions regarding possible beneficial or detrimental effects of training on the immune system in HIV-seropositive subjects.

REFERENCES

1. Fauci AS. Immunologic abnormalities in the acquired immunodeficiency syndrome (AIDS). Clin Res 1984; 32:491-499.
2. Fauci AS. The human immunodeficiency virus: infectivity and mechanisms of pathogenesis. Science 1988; 239:617-622.
3. Ullum H, Gotzsche PC, Victor J et al. Defective natural immunity: an early manifestation of human immunodeficiency virus infection. J Exp Med 1995; 182(3):789-799.
4. Hoffman-Goetz L, Pedersen BK. Exercise and the immune system: a model of the stress response? Immunol Today 1994; 15(8):382-7.
5. Ullum H, Palmo J, Halkjaer Kristensen J et al. The effect of acute exercise on lymphocyte subsets, natural killer cells, proliferative responses, and cytokines in HIV-seropositive persons. J Acquir Immune Defic Syndr 1994; 7(11):1122-1133.
6. Detels R, Visscher BR, Fahey JL et al. Predictors of clinical AIDS in young homosexual men in a high-risk area. Int J Epidemiol 1987; 16:271-276.
7. Moss AR, Bacchetti P, Osmond D et al. Seropositivity for HIV and the development of AIDS or AIDS related condition: three year followup of the San Francisco General Hospital cohort. Br Med J Clin Res Ed 1988; 296(6624):745-750.
8. Polk BF, Fox R, Brookmeyer R et al. Predictors of the acquired immunodeficiency syndrome developing in a cohort of seropositive homosexual men. N Engl J Med 1987; 316:61-66.
9. Safai B, Johnson KG, Myskowski PL et al. The natural history of Kaposi's sarcoma in the acquired immunodeficiency syndrome. Ann Intern Med 1985; 103:744-750.
10. Taylor J, Afrasiabi R, Fahey JL et al. Prognostically significant classification of immune changes in AIDS with Kaposi's sarcoma. Blood 1986; 67(3):666-671.

11. Anonymous Concorde: MRC/ANRS randomized double-blind controlled trial of immediate and deferred zidovudine in symptom-free HIV infection. Concorde Coordinating Committee. Lancet 1994; 343(8902):871-881.
12. Kovacs JA, Baseler M, Dewar RJ et al. Increases in CD4 T lymphocytes with intermittent courses of interleukin-2 in patients with human immunodeficiency virus infection. A preliminary study. N Engl J Med 1995; 332(9):567-575.
13. Taylor JM, Fahey JL, Detels R et al. CD4 percentage, CD4 number, and CD4:CD8 ratio in HIV infection: which to choose and how to use. J Acquir Immune Defic Syndr 1989; 2:114-124.
14. Doweiko JP. Hematologic aspects of HIV infection. AIDS 1993; 7:753-757.
15. Pedersen BK, Tvede N, Christensen LD et al. Natural killer cell activity in peripheral blood of highly trained and untrained persons. Int J Sports Med 1989; 10(2):129-131.
16. Tvede N, Steensberg J, Baslund B et al. Cellular immunity in highly trained elite racing cyclists during periods of training with high and low intensity. Scand J Med Sci Sports 1991; 1:163-6.
17. Nieman DC, Brendle D, Henson DA et al. Immune function in athletes versus nonathletes. Int J Sports Med 1995; 16(5):329-33.
18. Nieman DC, Buckley KS, Henson DA et al. Immune function in marathon runners versus sedentary controls. Med Sci Sports Exerc 1995; 27(7):986-992.
19. Oshida Y, Yamanouchi K, Hayamizu S et al. Effect of acute physical exercise on lymphocyte subpopulations in trained and untrained subjects. Int J Sports Med 1988; 9(2):137-140.
20. LaPerriere A, Antoni MH, Ironson G et al. Effects of aerobic exercise training on lymphocyte subpopulations. Int J Sports Med 1994; 15(Suppl 3):S127-S130.
21. Nieman DC, Henson DA, Gusewitch G et al. Physical activity and immune function in elderly women. Med Sci Sports Exerc 1993; 25(7):823-831.
22. Nieman DC, Nehlsen Cannarella SL, Markoff PA et al. The effects of moderate exercise training on natural killer cells and acute upper respiratory tract infections. Int J Sports Med 1990; 11(6):467-473.
23. Barnes CA, Forster MJ, Fleshner M et al. Exercise does not modify spatial memory, brain autoimmunity, or antibody response in aged F-344 rats. Neurobiol Aging 1991; 12(1):47-53.
24. Crist DM, Mackinnon LT, Thompson RF et al. Physical exercise increases natural cellular-mediated tumor cytotoxity in elderly women. Gerontology 1989; 35:66-71.

25. Nieman DC. Prolonged aerobic exercise, immune response, and risk of infection. In: Hoffman-Goetz L, ed. Exercise and Immune Function. New York: CRC Press, 1996:143-162.
26. Rigsby LW, Dishman RK, Jackson AW et al. Effects of exercise training on men seropositive for the human immunodeficiency virus-1. Med Sci Sports Exerc 1992; 24(1):6-12.
27. LaPerriere A, Antoni MH, Schneiderman N et al. Exercise Intervention Attenuates Emotional Distress and Killer Cell Decrements Following Notification of Positive Serologic Status for HIV-1. Biofeedback and Self-Regulation 1990; 15(3):229-242.
28. LaPerriere A, Fletcher MA, Antoni MH et al. Aerobic exercise training in an AIDS risk group. Int J Sports Med 1991; 12(Suppl 1):S53-57.
29. Birk TJ, MacArthur RD. Chronic exercise training maintains previously attained cardiopulmonary fitness in patients seropositive for human immunodeficiency virus type 1. Sports Med Train Rehab 1994; 5:1-6.
30. MacArthur RD, Levine SD, Birk TJ. Supervised exercise training improves cardiopulmonary fitness in HIV-infected persons. Med Sci Sports Exerc 1993; 25(6):684-8.
31. Ho DD, Neumann AU, Perelson AS et al. Rapid turnover of plasma virions and CD4 lymphocytes in HIV-1 infection. Nature 1995; 373(6510):123-126.
32. Wei X, Ghosh SK, Taylor ME et al. Viral dynamics in human immunodeficiency virus type 1 infection. Nature 1995; 373(6510): 117-122.

CHAPTER 9

Exercise and Infection

Bente Klarlund Pedersen

Without a doubt, exercise and to some degree training and fitness levels influence the concentration of immunocompetent cells in the circulating pool, the proportional distribution of lymphocyte subpopulations and the function of these cells. The important question is, however, to what degree are these immunological changes of clinical significance, that is does exercise influence our resistance to infectious diseases?

EXERCISE DURING POLIO INFECTION

During the acute phase of disease, rest has generally been considered beneficial, and patients are normally advised to stay in bed if they had fever. Support, based on modern scientific principles, for the benefits of rest in infectious diseases has been obtained during the present century.[1]

In the 1930s and 1940s, it was demonstrated that polio took a more serious course if patients had exercised during the early stages of the disease. The idea that physical exercise might influence the clinical outcome of poliomyelitis was based on sporadic reports of a great physical exertion prior to the onset of severe paralysis. One of the first reports was by Collier et al[2] in 1927. In 1930, Limper et al[3] found that exhausting exercise preceded the onset of the disease in patients who were victims of the San Francisco Epidemic of 1930. One of the patients, who had been ill in bed for 2 days with vague symptoms, then improved sufficiently to participate in an unusually hard-fought football game. Within a few hours he developed symptoms of poliomyelitis, which terminated in extensive paralysis and death from respiratory failure. In 1932, Voss et al[4] reported a case of ascending poliomyelitis in a 17-year-old girl after a tennis match. In the same year, Bremer[5] reported a case of the disease in a student following a vigorous mountain climb. Tebbutt and Helms[6] in Australia noted that exhausting exercise had immediately preceded the onset of the disease in several patients who subsequently developed severe and widespread paralysis.

Despite many sporadic reports on vigorous exercise preceding paralysis, these did not provide any information on a possible causal relationship. However, a striking phenomenon reported by Howe and Bodian[7] stimulated Russell[8,9] to investigate the influence of exercise statistically. Howe and Bodian[7] made the interesting observation that if the anterior horn cell was engaged in regenerating its neuroaxon, that is, if the peripheral nerve originating in these cells had been sectioned a few days previously, these anterior cells were then quite immune to experimental infection with virus. Based on this, it was by no means impossible, that physical activity at a certain stage of disease might alter the motor neuron physiology in such a way as to influence its susceptibility to infection.

Russell[8,9] studied the effect of physical exercise during the preparalytic period. In total he reported 100 cases of poliomyelitis studying the initial symptoms in details. The patients were questioned about their early meningitis-like symptoms consisting of pain in the head, neck, dorsal, lumbar or sacral spine. Physical activity of any kind during the paralytic stage increased the danger of severe paralysis, whereas complete physical rest during the whole of the preparalytic stage protected the patient from severe paralysis.

These observations concerning poliomyelitis were later confirmed in other epidemiological studies, as well as in experimental animal studies. Hargreaves[10] analyzed 30 cases of poliomyelitis and confirmed the previous findings by Russell[8,9] that physical exercise in the preparalytic phase was associated with grave prognoses. Furthermore, he suggested that severe mental stress such as driving a car over long distances, appeared to be equally disastrous.

Horstmann studied 411 patients with poliomyelitis from three epidemics.[11] It was found that physical activity performed after the second phase or major illness was associated with a significant increase in incidence and severity of subsequent paralysis. Furthermore, a higher percentage of nonparalytic cases was found, if patients gave a history of bed rest or minimal activity during the early stages of the major illness.

The finding that physical activity worsened the clinical outcome of poliomyelitis has been experimentally substantiated in experiments with monkeys[12] and mice.[13] Levinson et al[12] showed higher incidence of paralysis in monkeys, who performed exhausting exercise during the incubation period of experimental poliomyelitis developed compared to controls. Histologic examination of sections of the brain and cord of test and control animals disclosed characteristic changes of poliomyelitis which in general correlated in degree of severity with clinical observations. The use of monkeys limited the numbers of animals in the experiment. The availability of a mice model in the study by Rosenbaum and Harford[13] permitted the use of relatively larger numbers of animals (n = 551). Mice were forced to run during the day preceding and daily subsequent to the intracerebral injection of experimental poliomyelitis. The incidence of the disease as measured both by paralysis and by death was greater in the exercised animals than in the resting controls.

EXERCISE AND HEPATITIS INFECTION

Since the end of World War II, rest has been considered essential for the treatment of infectious hepatitis and the current medical opinion has been that a patient should not be allowed to resume normal physical activity until the liver function is normal. However, in contrast to the studies on poliomyelitis, several studies show that physical exercise does not worsen the disease outcome of hepatitis. Although the finding of fulminant hepatitis in five patients, who had all undertaken vigorous exercise during the early stages of the illness, gave rise to the suspicion that exercise had worsened the disease outcome.[14] Several studies on large number of patients, including controlled studies, found exercise in relation to hepatitis to be safe.[15-18]

Chalmers et al[15] showed that ad libitum ward privileges with only 1 hour of rest after each meal did not adversely affect recovery as compared with patients treated with strict bed rest. Moreover, the amount of activity between onset of symptoms and hospitalization was unrelated to eventual recovery, and participation in a vigorous reconditioning program after normal liver function had been attained was not associated with either clinical or biochemical relapse.

Repsher and Freebern[17] compared the effect of strenuous exercise on recovery time in 199 American servicemen in Vietnam with infectious hepatitis to that in 199 patients with infectious hepatitis treated in the customary fashion. The exercise group was started on the program of strenuous exercise for approximately 3 hours daily at the time their symptoms were considered to be slight, irrespective of the degree of liver-function abnormality. There were no differences between the two groups regarding elevation of serum bilirubin or duration of disease. Furthermore, strenuous exercise compared to slight activity at the time of onset illness did not influence the disease outcome.

Nelson et al[16] studied 80 patients and did not find that exercise inhibited sustained recovery in the patients even though many had been very active during the acute illness. Nefzger and Chalmers[18] performed a 10 year followup study on the effects of diet and rest on the outcome of hepatitis. It was found that the forced intake of high-protein diet shortened the period for acute illness by about 20%, but rest did not seem to have any influence on the acute disease or the longterm outcome.

From these studies it can be concluded that strenuous exercise during the early reconvalescence of viral hepatitis does not cause relapse of any clinical significance or prolong recovery time. In fact exercise does not seem to be harmful, even in the acute phase.

EXERCISE AND MYOCARDITIS

One major reason why doctors advise against performing vigorous exercise during acute infections is the potential of supervening myocarditis.[1] The effect of exercise in the acute phase of Coxsackie B virus myocarditis has been investigated in several experimental studies.[19-21]

Acute exercise causes increased viral replication, inflammation and necrosis in the myocardium. In the study by Gatmaitan et al,[20] 14-day-old mice were studied. In mice infected with murine coxsackievirus B-3, swimming in the initial phase of the infection, increased mortality from 5.5-50%. Many of the affected mice died of congestive heart failure while swimming. Their hearts were dilated and necrotic and mean heart to body weight increased. Virtually every myocardial fiber showed pathological change as opposed to 1/4-1/2 of myocardial involvement in the nonexercising mice. When swimming was initiated 9 days after virus inoculation, while virus replication was waning, mortality increased only 13.8% over nonexercised controls. The findings by Gatmaitan et al[20] is in accordance with previous findings showing that coxsackievirus infections have been initiated by immunosuppression induced by corticosteroids[22] and lends support to the hypothesis that intense exercise induces immunosuppression of clinical importance.

Ilback et al[19] inoculated mice with coxsackievirus B-3 and exercised them to exhaustion up to 48 hours after inoculation. Exercise at the same time as virus inoculation did not influence the myocardial damage, whereas exercise at 48 hours after the inoculation increased the myocardial damage significantly. In this study, lethality was not influenced by exercise. The exercise-associated increased myocardial inflammation was related to a decreased number of cells expressing major histocompatibility complex class II, such as macrophages. Thus the extent of tissue damage in these mice may be related to decreased macrophage mobilization followed by increased destruction of the myocardium, possibly mediated by cytotoxic T cells.

Myocarditis may result in either no symptoms, vague symptoms or frank symptoms such as chest pain, discomfort, dyspnea or irregular heart rhythm. The finding that myocarditis can occur without clinical symptoms is in line with the finding of active myocarditis in 1% of unselected autopsies performed during a 10-year period.[23] Sudden death in the acute phase of symptomatic or asymptomatic myocarditis is a well-known phenomenon,[24] but myocarditis accounts for only 10% of sudden unexpected cardiac deaths in young sportsmen.

Recently, Swedish orienteering has been struck by an accumulation of sudden deaths. Sixteen young Swedish orienteers suffered from sudden unexpected cardiac deaths from 1979 to 1992.[25] No sudden unexpected deaths among young orienteers have occurred since 1992. Histopathological evaluation showed active myocarditis in five cases,[25] arrhytmogenic right ventricular dysplasia-like alterations in four cases; the remaining seven cases could not be classified into either of the previous groups. Tissue sampling which allowed testing for a variety of microorganisms was performed in only the two recent fatalities; in one of these cases, polymerase chain reaction (PCR) with the primers directed to the rRNA gene of *Chlamydia pneumoniae* was found in the heart and lungs, but not in specimens from several other organs.[25,26] All cultures and PCR for other microorganisms were negative.

It is not possible to explain the accumulation of deaths among Swedish orienteers. Such a death rate did not occur within other endurance sports in Sweden during the same period of time. Chlamydia pneumonia is likely to be the cause of one of the cases who had suffered from prolonged respiratory tract infection prior to death and in whom active myocarditis was found. *Chlamydia pneumoniae* is a common pathogen, which normally causes upper respiratory tract infection (URTI) and eventually pneumonia. Approximately 20% of the Scandinavian population has antibodies against Chlamydia pneumonia, showing that infection with *Chlamydia pneumoniae* is very common. One theory is, however, that postexercise immunosuppression allows relatively harmless microorganisms such as Coxsackie B virus and *Chlamydia pneumonia* to invade the host, actively replicate and spread from the upper respiratory tract to the circulation, the lungs and the heart. Thereby, relatively harmless microorganisms behave like highly virulent microorganisms.

EXERCISE AND OTHER INFECTIONS

In 1922, Nicholls and Spaeth[27] reported that 80% of sedentary guinea pigs died after exposure to type I pneumococcus, whereas animals given acute exercise prior to inoculation showed only a 20% fatality rate. The protective effect of artificially induced fatigue was found in both white and pigmented rats and occurred whether fatigue preceded or followed the pneumococcal infection, but was distinctly more effective in the case of exercise before injection. Exercise in mice infected with *Toxoplasma gondii* did not significantly alter the disease outcome, although a more rapid recovery was associated with exercise as levels of serum tumor necrosis factor (TNF) were reduced.[28]

Moderate exercise in mice during infection with influenza or tularemia counteracted the infection-induced decrease in the activities of glycolytic and oxidative enzymes in tularemia, but lethality and bacterial counts in the spleen were unaffected. However, exhaustive exercises in combination with influenza increased lethality.[29]

Mice trained on running wheels and then injected with *Salmonella typhimurium* had a significantly higher survival rate than sedentary mice and it was suggested that this was related to an exercise-induced increase in the level of interleukin (IL)-1 and a concomitant acute phase response.[30] The same results were obtained in influenza-infected mice, thus physically conditioned mice showed lower mortality rate.[29] This might be related to the fact that the myocardial protein-degrading effect of influenza did not occur with preconditioning, and oxidative tissue enzyme activities decreased less. Ilback et al[31] showed that a 4 week training program in rats with gradually increasing swimming time prior to infection with pneumococcus caused no protection from lethality, but the catabolic response was less pronounced.

From the above mentioned studies, it is clear that the effects of exercise stress on disease lethality varies with the type and time that it is performed. In general, it is shown that exercise or training before infection has either no effect or decreases morbidity and mortality, whereas exercise during the infection has either no effect or increases severity of infection. The importance of timing was shown in a study on the influence of exercise stress on susceptibility to *Streptococcus pneumoniae* and *Francisella tularensis* infections. It was shown that strenuous exercise immediately before infection drastically reduced susceptibility to either of the bacteria, whereas a similar bout of exercise performed after infection increased disease-related mortality in both diseases.[32]

EXERCISE AND UPPER RESPIRATORY TRACT INFECTIONS

A large proportion of runners claim to have fewer respiratory infections since they started running.[33] However, based on anecdotal information a general feeling has been that while regular training promotes resistance to URTI, severe exertion, especially when coupled with mental stress, places athletes at increased risk for URTI.[34,35] During the past decade several epidemiological studies on exercise and URTI have been reported.

Peters and Bateman[36] carried out a prospective study of the incidence of symptoms of URTI in 150 randomly selected runners who took part in the 1982 Two Oceans Marathon in Cape Town and compared them with the incidence in individually matched controls who did not run. Runners were questioned on the day before and 2 weeks after the race. Symptoms of URTI occurred in 33.3% of runners compared with 15.3% of controls and were most common in those who achieved the faster race times. Thus, the frequency of URTI reported was inversely related to the time taken to complete the race (Fig. 9.1) and 47% of the faster runners experienced symptoms.

Linde[37] studied URTI over a 1 year period among 44 elite orienteers. A nonathletic group matched for sex and age, and occupational distribution, acted as a control group with regard to disease frequency. The orienteers had 2.5 URTI per year on average against 1.7 in the control group ($p < 0.05$). The length of disease was 7.9 days and 6.4 days, respectively (not significant).

Nieman et al[38] studied the incidence of infectious episodes in 273 runners during a 2 month training period prior to a 5 km, 10 km or half-marathon race. In addition the effect of the race experience on infectious episodes was studied. Only 6.8% of the runners preparing for the half-marathon race reported becoming sick with the flu versus 17.9% of the 5 km and 10 km runners ($p = 0.067$). Thus, this study showed a trend that runners with a more serious commitment to regular exercise had less infectious episodes.

The largest epidemiological study on exercise and URTI was performed by Nieman et al[39] who researched the incidence of URTI in a group of 2311 marathon runners who took part in the 1987

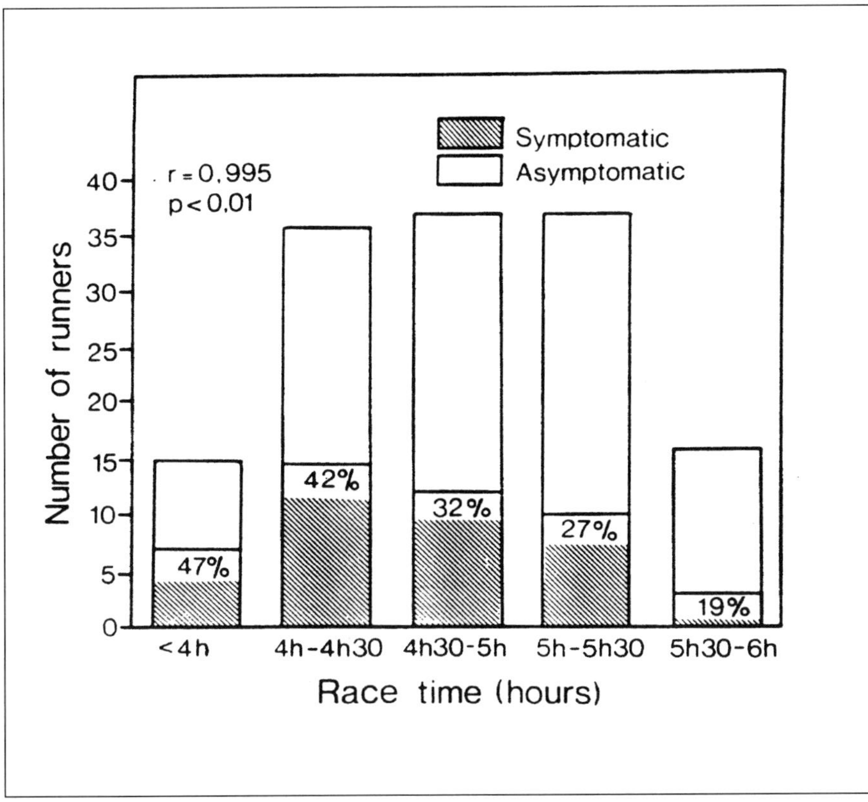

Fig. 9.1. Distribution of symptomatic and asymptomatic runners according to time taken to complete the race (N = 141). Reprinted with permission from Peters EM et al, South Afr Med J 1983; 64:582-584.

Los Angeles Marathon race. It was found that 12.9% of Los Angeles Marathon participants reported an infectious episode during the week following the race in comparison to only 2.2% of similarly experienced runners who had applied but did not participate (for reasons other than sickness). Controlling for important demographic and training data by using logistic regression, it was determined that the odds were six to one in favor of sickness for the marathon race participants versus the nonparticipating runners.

Heath et al[40] examined the illness pattern in a cohort of 530 male and female runners during a period of 1 year. The 530 runners reported a total of 643 URTIs for the year and 66% had at least one URTI. Controlling for various confounding variables using a model of logistic regression it was shown that the odds ratio was two to one for URTI for persons running more than 1388 miles per year.

In a prospective study of URTI in 12-year-old children engaged in sports, there was, however, no difference in infection rates between the sports participants and controls during the course of a year.[41]

There are very few studies comparing URTI in large groups of moderately active individuals. However, two randomized experimental trials using small numbers of subjects have provided important data in support of the viewpoint that moderate physical activity may reduce URTI symptomatology. A study that examined 36 women who performed a 15 week walking program (45 minutes of walking, 5 days per week) reported significantly fewer days with URTI symptoms during the 15 week study than in the control group (5.1 vs. 10.8 days). The number of separate URTI did not vary between groups, but the number of URTI symptom days per incident was lower in the exercising group (Fig. 9.2).[42] In a randomized controlled study of elderly women, 67-85 years old, the incidence of the common cold during a 12 week period in the fall was measured to be the lowest in highly conditioned subjects who exercised moderately each day for about 1.5 hours (8%). Elderly subjects who walked 40 minutes, five times per week had an incidence of 21%, compared with 50% for the sedentary control group.[43] This study clearly showed that elderly women not engaging in cardiorespiratory exercise are more likely to experience an URTI during the fall season than those who do not exercise regularly.

Based on the above mentioned epidemiological studies a relationship between exercise and URTI has been modeled in the form of a "J" curve (Fig. 9.2). This model suggests that while the risk of URTI may decrease below that of sedentary individuals when one engages in moderate exercise training, the risk may rise above average during periods of excessive amount of high-intensity exercise.[44]

INTERVENTION STUDIES

Intervention studies have been carried out based on a theory that competitive distance running resulted in alterations in the

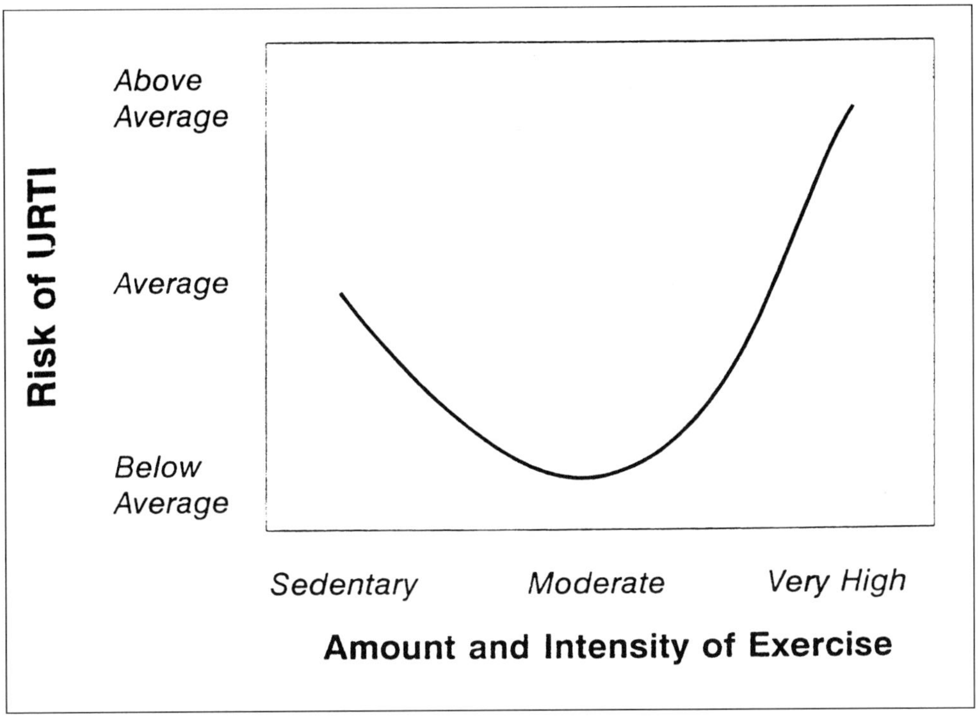

Fig. 9.2. "J"-shaped model of relationship between varying amounts of exercise and risk of upper respiratory tract infection (URTI). This model suggests that moderate exercise may lower risk of respiratory infection while excessive amounts may increase risk. Reprinted with permission from Nieman DC et al, Med Sci Sports Exerc 1994; 26(2):128-39.

hormonal milieu that, in turn, affects free radical production rates and hence immunological function. Anti-oxidants may in theory neutralize the reactive species which are produced by neutrophilic leukocytes during phagocytosis.[45,46] It is generally accepted that ascorbate is an important anti-oxidant in the blood and interstitial fluids, and that its primary target in promoting immunocompetence appears to be the phagocyte, particularly the neutrophil.[47]

Using a double blind placebo design, Peters[48] reported that the URTI incidence was 68% after 90 km Comrades Ultramarathon. This was significantly more than in the vitamin C supplementation group, where only 33% reported URTI when taking a 600 mg Vitamin C supplementation daily for 3 weeks prior to the race. In another study, Peters et al[49] found that vitamin A supplementation had an insignificant effect on the incidence of URTI in marathoners.

PRACTICAL GUIDELINES

What to tell athletes about exercising with an URTI? It is difficult to determine early on that an "URTI" is only a rhinovirus, and not an incipient mycoplasma pneumonia, chlamydia pneumonia or Coxsackie B virus infection. Therefore, the general advice is to rest when sick. This can be modified when the symptoms have lasted for a day or two and are strictly "above the neck" (stuffy or runny nose, sneezing, watery eyes, scratchy throat and no fever). However, when symptoms are "below the neck" (aching muscles, hacking cough, nausea, vomiting, diarrhea) the advice is definitely to abstain training.[50]

CONCLUSION

Exercise or training before inoculation of an infectious agent tends to decrease susceptibility to infectious diseases. This may be related to the finding of slightly better resting levels of the immune system in trained subjects compared to untrained. Moderate exercise during the infection does not influence the outcome of the disease; in theory, light exercise may accelerate the clearing of the microorganisms by boosting the immune response but this has not been found. Exhaustive exercise during an infection, generally causes increased severity of infection and lethality. This is probably related to exercise-associated immunosuppression which allows more rapid replication of microorganisms and support the "open window" theory. However, the nature of the microorganisms and the localization of the infection may play a role. Friman and Ilback[1] stress the point that those examples (poliomyelitis and myocarditis), where exercise seems to worsen the clinical disease, are typified by the location of the infectious process within a tissue or organ that is mechanically or metabolically active as a result of exercise. The higher incidence of URTI following intense exercise may not just be attributable to the impairment of natural immunity but the physical effects of cold and dry air on local mucosal defenses may directly inhibit the secretory immune system. The finding of a decreased incidence of URTI in individuals who perform moderate training is in accordance with the finding that moderate exercise stimulates the immune system, whereas intense exercise suppresses the immune response.

References

1. Friman G, Ilback NG. Exercise and infection—interaction, risks and benefits. Scand J Med Sci Sports 1992; 2:177-89.
2. Collier J. Lancet 1927; 1:321.
3. Limper MA, Thelander HE, Shaw EB. Poliomyelitis in adults: Report of 60 cases. J Prev Med 1931; 5:475-489.
4. Voss G. Ein fall von pyeliomyelitis ascendens acutissima. Deutsche med Wehnschr 1931; 58:1882-1883.
5. Bremer FW. Ueber das klinische Bild und die Therapie der Heine-Medinschen Krankheit beim Erwachsenen. Deutsches Srch f klin Med 1932; 173:58-67.
6. Tebbutt AH, Helms K. Report of the epidemic of poliomyelitis in New South Wales. Med J Austr 1933; 1:43-60.
7. Howe HA, Bodian D. Neural Mechanisms in Poliomyelitis. New York:1942.
8. Russel WR. Poliomyelitis. The preparalytic stage, and the effect of physical activity on the severity of paralysis. Br Med J 1947; 2:1023-1028.
9. Russel WR. Paralytic Poliomyelitis. The early symptoms and the effct of physical activity on the course of the disease. Br Med J 1949; 1:465-471.
10. Hargreaves ER. Poliomyelitis. Effect of exertion during the preparalytic stage. Br Med J 1948; 2:1021-1022.
11. Horstmann DM. Acute Poliomyelitis. Relation of physical activity at the time of onset to the course of the disease. JAMA 1950; 142:236-241.
12. Levinson S, Miltzer A, Lewin P. Effect of fatigue, chilling and mechanical trauma on resistance to experimental poliomyelitis. Am J Hygiene 1945; 42:204-312.
13. Rosenbaum HE, Harford CG. Effect of Fatigue on Susceptibility of Mice to Poliomyelitis. Proc Soc Exp Biol Med 1953; 83:678-681.
14. Krikler DM, Zilberg B. Activity and hepatitis. Lancet 1966; 2(472):1046-1047.
15. Chalmers T. The treatment of acute infectios hepatitis. Controlled studies of the effects of diet, rest and physical reconditioning on the acute course of the disease and on the incidence of relapses and residual abnormalities. J Clin Invest 1955; 34:1163-1235.
16. Nelson RS, Sprinz H, Colbert JW et al. Effects of physical exercise on recovery frem hepatitis. Am J Med 1954; 16:780-789.
17. Repsher LH, Freebern RK. Effects of early and vigorous exercise on recovery from infectious hepatitis. N Engl J Med 1969; 281(25):1393-1396.
18. Nefzger MD, Chalmers TC. The Treatment of Acute Infectious Hepatitis. A Ten-year followup study of the effects of diet and rest. Am J Physiol 1963; 35:299-309.

19. Ilback NG, Fohlman J, Friman G. Exercise in coxsackie B3 myocarditis: effects on heart lymphocyte subpopulations and the inflammatory reaction. Am Heart J 1989; 117(6):1298-1302.
20. Gatmaitan BG, Chanson JL, Lerner AM. Agumentation of the virulence of murine coxackievirus B-3 myocardiopathy by exercise. J Exp Med 1970; 131:1121-1136.
21. Reyes M. Proc Soc Exp Biol Med 1976; 151:333-338.
22. Kilbourne ED, Wilson CB, Perrier D. The induction of gross myocardial lesions by coxsackie (pleurodynia) virus and cortisone. J Clin Invest 1956; 35:362-366.
23. Gravanis MB, Sternby NH. Incidence of myocarditis. A 10-year autopsy study from Malmo, Sweden. Arch Pathol Lab Med 1991; 115(4):390-392.
24. Karjalainen J. Clinical diagnosis of myocarditis and dilated cardiomyopathy. Scand J Infect Dis Suppl 1993; 88:33-43.
25. Wesslen L, Påhlson C, Linquist O et al. An increase in sudden unexpected cardiac deaths among young Swedish orienteers during 1979-1992. Eur Heart J 1996; 17:902-910.
26. Wesslen L, Pahlson C, Friman G et al. Myocarditis caused by *Chlamydia pneumoniae* (TWAR) and sudden unexpected death in a Swedish elite orienteer. Lancet 1992; 340(8816):427-428.
27. Nicholls EE, Spaeth RA. The relation between fatigue and the susceptibility of guinea pigs to infections of type I pneumococcus. Am J Hygiene 1922; 2:527-535.
28. Chao CC, Strgar F, Tsang M et al. Effects of swimming exercise on the pathogenesis of acute murine *Toxoplasma gondii* Me49 infection. Clin Immunol Immunopathol 1992; 62(2):220-226.
29. Ilback NG, Friman G, Beisel WR et al. Sequential metabolic alterations in the myocardium during influenza and tularemia in mice. Infect Immun 1984; 45(2):491-497.
30. Cannon JG, Kluger MJ. Exercise enhances survival rate in mice infected with *Salmonella typhimurium.* Proc Soc Exp Biol Med 1984; 175(4):518-521.
31. Ilback NG, Friman G, Crawford DJ et al. Effects of training on metabolic responses and performance capacity in *Streptococcus pneumoniae* infected rats. Med Sci Sports Exerc 1991; 23(4):422-427.
32. Ilback NG, Crawford DJ, Neufeld HA et al. Does exercise stress alter susceptibility to bacterial infections? Ups J Med Sci 1991; 96(1):63-68.
33. Green RL, Kaplan SS, Rabin BS et al. Immune function in marathon runners. Ann Allergy 1981; 47(2):73-75.
34. Fitzgerald L. Overtraining increases the susceptibility to infection. Int J Sports Med 1991; 12(Suppl 1):S5-8.

35. Nieman DC. Exercise, infection, and immunity. Int J Sports Med 1994; 15 Suppl 3:S131-S141.
36. Peters EM, Bateman ED. Ultramaraton running and upper respiratory tract infections. An epidemiological survey. South Afr Med J 1983; 64:582-584.
37. Linde F. Running and upper respiratory tract infections. Scand J Sports Sci 1987; 9:21-23.
38. Nieman DC, Johanssen LM, Lee JW. Infectious episodes in runners before and after a roadrace. J Sports Med Phys Fit 1989; 29(3):289-296.
39. Nieman DC, Johanssen LM, Lee JW et al. Infectious episodes in runners before and after the Los Angeles Marathon. J Sports Med Phys Fit 1990; 30(3):316-328.
40. Heath GW, Ford ES, Craven TE et al. Exercise and the incidence of upper respiratory tract infections. Med Sci Sports Exerc 1991; 23(2):152-157.
41. Osterback L, Qvarnberg Y. A prospective study of respiratory infections in 12-year-old children actively engaged in sports. Acta Paediatr Scand 1987; 76(6):944-949.
42. Nieman DC, Nehlsen Cannarella SL, Markoff PA et al. The effects of moderate exercise training on natural killer cells and acute upper respiratory tract infections. Int J Sports Med 1990; 11(6):467-473.
43. Nieman DC, Henson DA, Gusewitch G et al. Physical activity and immune function in elderly women. Med Sci Sports Exerc 1993; 25(7):823-831.
44. Nieman DC. Exercise, upper respiratory tract infection, and the immune system. Med Sci Sports Exerc 1994; 26(2):128-39.
45. Babior BM. Oxidants from phagocytes: agents of defense and destruction. Blood 1984; 64: (5):959-966.
46. Hemila H. Vitamin C and the common cold. Br J Nutr 1992; 67(1):3-16.
47. Anderson R, Lukey PT. A biological role for ascorbate in the selective neutralization of extracellular phagocyte-derived oxidants. Ann NY Acad Sci 1987; 498:229-247.
48. Peters EM, Goetzsche JM, Grobbelaar B et al. Vitamin C supplementation reduces the incidence of postrace symptoms of upper-respiratory-tract infection in ultramarathon runners. Am J Clin Nutr 1993; 57(2):170-174.
49. Peters EM, Cambell A, Pawley L. Vitamin A fails to increase resistance to upper respiratory in distance runners. S Afr J Sports Med 1992; 7:3-7.
50. Eichner ER. Infection, immunity, and exercise: What to tell patients? Phys Sportsmed 1993; 21(1):125-35.

CHAPTER 10

Nutrition, Age and Immunity in Exercise

Bente Klarlund Pedersen and Helle Bruunsgaard

The relationship between nutritional factors and resistance to infections has generated considerable interest over the past several decades. In industrialized countries, the relationship between nutrition and immunity is of special interest in elderly subjects, since it is known that age-related immunodeficiency is aggravated in malnourished subjects. In theory, it is possible that the exercise-induced immunological changes can be modulated by nutritional factors and that dietary factors influence resting levels of the immune system. Furthermore, aging is associated with a suppression in the normal function of the immune system which may influence the ability to respond to physical stress. Nutritional supplementation may partly revert this immune senescence.

On this background a short review will be given on the influence of protein-energy malnutrition, lipid metabolism and vitamin deficiency on the immune system. Furthermore, the potential protective role of functional food in restoring age-related and exercise-induced immunosuppression will be discussed.

PROTEIN-ENERGY MALNUTRITION

It has been suggested that malnutrition is the most common cause of immunodeficiency worldwide.[1] Mild to moderate undernutrition is not uncommon even in industrialized countries. The

Exercise Immunology, edited by Bente Klarlund Pedersen. © 1997 R.G. Landes Company.

incidence of nutritional deficiencies is higher in certain at-risk groups including certain age-groups, e.g., low-birth weight infants, pregnant and nursing mothers and the elderly. Malnutrition is also related to poverty, illiteracy and lack of nutrition education.

Several epidemiological studies have documented the adverse effect of protein-energy malnutrition on morbidity and mortality. Thus, a significant correlation between protein-energy malnutrition and risk of death from infectious diseases was found in rural India.[2]

In another interesting study Victora, et al[3] studied the synergism between nutritional status and hospital admissions due to diarrhea in southern Brazil and found that malnutrition was a more important risk factor for pneumonia than for diarrhea, whereas diarrhea was a stronger predictor of malnutrition than was pneumonia—the association being strongest in the first two years of life.

Soldiers undergoing a rigorous training, which include severe food restriction as well as other stressors, suffer from increased incidence of infections.[4]

In protein-energy malnutrition, most of the host defense mechanisms are impaired (Table 10.1).[5,6] The delayed cutaneous hypersensitivity responses to several recall antigens are markedly depressed in moderate deficiencies and complete anergy is observed in severe protein-energy malnutrition. The skin reactions are restored after appropriate nutritional therapy for several weeks or months.[7]

The concentration of $CD4^+$ cells is decreased in malnourished and a moderate reduction in the number of $CD8^+$ cells has been reported.[8,9] The serum antibody responses are generally intact in protein-energy malnutrition, but the antibody affinity was found to be decreased in malnourished patients.[10]

Hoffman-Goetz et al[11,12] showed that malnutrition in rats altered the ability of T cells to respond appropriately to cytokines. Furthermore, the production of interleukin (IL)-1, IL-2 and interferon (IFN)-γ is decreased in protein-energy malnutrition. Complement is an essential opsonin and the levels and activity of most complement components are decreased. Thereby the phagocytosis is also affected in protein-energy malnutrition.[13,14]

In a study by Kono et al,[15] phagocytic function was found to be higher in leukocytes from athletes compared with those from

Table 10.1. Immune alterations with protein-energy malnutrition and their sequelae

T cells	CD4 concentration↓ CD8 concentration↓ DTH↓
B cells	Antibody affinity↓
Monocytes	Phagocytic function↓
Cytokines	IL-1 production↓ IL-2 production↓ IFNγ production↓
Complement	Level and activity of complement components↓
Hormones	Corticosterone↑
Sequelae	Increased incidence of infections

controls before initiation of caloric restriction. After a weight reduction of 4% in 2 weeks at 65% of the usual caloric consumption during training, it was found that weight loss significantly depressed phagocytic function. Therefore, the exercise-induced enhancement of phagocyte function was antagonized by food restriction or weight loss. An animal study by Filteau et al[16] found some evidence for the hypothesis that exercise can prevent undernutrition-induced immunodepression in female mice. Immunodepression induced by undernutrition was only reflected by decreased spleen and thymus weight and elevated corticosterone level. Exercise did not enhance any of these indices of immune function in the ad libitum fed mice. However, exercise in the underfed mice significantly attenuated the decrease in spleen (but not thymus) weight, attenuated the elevation in corticosterone and enhanced the proliferative response.

In her recent review on interactive effects of exercise and food restriction on the immune system, Conn[17] stresses the point that most animal experiments have used underfeeding of the same diet given to the control animals rather than restricting the energy intake while ensuring adequacy of essential nutrients. It is possible that the effect on the immune system of undernutrition without malnutrition combined with exercise differs from that observed in studies on effects of malnutrition and exercise.

Dietary deficiency or stress-induced suppression of selected amino acids such as glutamine may in theory cause suppression of the lymphocyte function. In vitro studies have clearly shown that glutamine is required for optimal growth of lymphocytes and monocytes, for the cytotoxic activity of lymphokine activated killer (LAK) cells and the production of IL-2, IL-6 and IFN-γ.[18,19] It has also been shown that the glutamine concentration declines following intense exercise and other physical stress forms,[18,20,21] but it remains to be shown whether a causal relationship exists between low plasma-glutamine concentration and suppressed cellular immune function.

VITAMINS

Vitamin B_6 is the collective term for the metabolically and functionally related pyridoxines. They are involved in the metabolism of protein and cellular proliferation.[22,23] A number of animal studies have reported that cell-mediated immunity is profoundly affected by vitamin B_6 deficiency. Thus, it has been shown that delayed type hypersensitivity, mixed lymphocyte reaction, lymphocyte proliferation and cytotoxic responses were depressed in vitamin B_6 deficiency.[24-26]

A recent study was designed to study the effects of isoniazid on the immune system. Healthy volunteers were given isoniazid and pyridoxin for 30 days, while the control group was only given pyridoxin. Pyridoxin was given to avoid neurological side effects and the study was not designed to evaluate possible effects of pyridoxin on the cell-mediated immune response as the study did not include a nontreatment group. However, it was found that pyridoxin stimulated the phytohemagglutinin (PHA)-induced proliferative response and the natural killer (NK) cell activity.[27] These findings were in accordance with previous findings by Chandra and Sudhakaran (Table 10.2).[28]

Vitamin E deficiency is rare in human beings, and most studies on vitamin E deficiency have been performed in animals. These studies have shown that vitamin E is essential for normal function of the immune system and that deficiency of vitamin E is associated

Table 10.2. Immune alterations with vitamin deficiency and their sequelae

Vitamin B_6 deficiency	T cells	DTH↓ MLR↓ Proliferative responses↓
Vitamin E deficiency	Neutrophils	Chemotaxis↓ Bactericidal activity↓ Oxidative metabolic responses↓
Vitamin C deficiency	Neutrophils Macrophages	Bactericidal capacity↓ Bactericidal capacity↓
Vitamin A deficiency	T lymphocytes Mucosa	Proliferative response↓ Increased bacterial adherence

with a decline of the immune response, whereas higher than required amounts have stimulatory effects.[29]

The few immunological studies on vitamin E deficient humans, include newborn infants, pre-term infants, children with chronic cholestasis and glutathione-deficient newborn infants. The depressed neutrophil chemotaxis, bactericidal activity and oxidative metabolic responses in these patients were restored after vitamin E supplementation (Table 10.2).[30,31]

The role of vitamin C in phagocyte function has been recognized. Moderately severe deficiency is associated with decreased bactericidal capacity of neutrophils and macrophages, whereas cell-mediated immunity and antibody production are relatively unaffected (Table 10.2).[32]

Vitamin A has been known as an anti-infective vitamin and deficiency in vitamin A results in decreased lymphocyte proliferation and increased bacterial adherence to respiratory epithelial cells (Table 10.2).[1,33,34]

Supplementary studies have been performed to test the efficacy of anti-oxidant supplements in enhancing resistance to upper respiratory tract infections (URTI) following intense, long-lasting exercise such as a marathon. Peters et al[35] conducted a double-blind placebo-controlled study on runners and their matched nonrunning controls participating in the 1990 Comrades Marathon. Supplementing with 600 mg vitamin C daily for 3 weeks prior to the 90 km race resulted in a significantly reduced incidence of postrace upper respiratory tract infection symptoms when compared to the incidence amongst the runners receiving placebo. The vitamin C supplemented group 33% reported symptoms of URTI as opposed to an incidence of 68% in the runners receiving placebo. Vitamin C had no effect on the incidence of URTI symptoms in the sedentary group.

Supplementing with vitamin A had no significant effect on the incidence of URTI in distance runners.[36] There is accumulating evidence showing that vitamin E in combination with vitamin C is the most effective way to stop the chain of free radicals produced in the cells.[37,38]

Interesting studies which examine the influence of vitamin E on exercise-induced neutrocytosis[39] and the acute phase response[40] have been performed. The changes in circulating neutrophils in young and older men in response to 45 minutes of downhill running exercise were investigated.[39] In the young subjects circulating neutrophils rose after exercise, reaching peak levels after 6 hours. The response was unaffected by vitamin E supplementation. However, in older subjects vitamin E inhibited the postexercise rise in circulating neutrophils.[39] In another study the same group investigated the influence of muscle damaging eccentric exercise on in vitro production and plasma concentrations of cytokines after previous intake of vitamin E for 48 hours.[40] In this double blind placebo controlled study it was found that endotoxin-induced secretion of IL-1β was augmented 154% in cells obtained from the placebo subjects after exercise. However, no significant exercise-related changes were observed in cells from the vitamin E supplemented subjects. Vitamin E had no influence on the exercise-induced enhancement of the secretion of TNF-α, but vitamin E did reduce the IL-6 production.

LIPIDS

The fatty acid composition of lymphocytes, monocytes and splenocytes can be modified by dietary fats by which the fluidity and the structure of the cell membranes are altered. This may be one of the mechanisms by which the dietary fats can either increase or decrease the activity of these cells.[41,42]

Another important mechanism regarding the interaction between lipids and the immune system is the relationship between lipid composition in the cellular pool and eicosanoid synthesis. All immunocompetent cells are able to synthesize eicosanoids from polyunsaturated fatty acids (PUFA). Which eicosanoids are synthesized depends upon the availability of precursors of n-6 and n-3 PUFA in the cellular phospholipid pool.[43] The amount of PUFA released on an intracellular level, as well as the rate of eicosanoid synthesis is determined by the activity of phospholipases as long as there is no fatty acids deficiency.[44]

The clinical relevance of the various PUFA is based on the potential for modification of prostaglandin and leukotriene synthesis. n-6 and n-3 are precursors of eicosanoids (i.e., prostaglandins, leukotrienes and thromboxanes) of different series. Macrophages appear to be one of the major immune cell sources that release eicosanoids in response to inflammatory stimuli. With respect to eicosanoid synthesis, linoleic acid, an essential n-6 fatty acid, serves as the primary source for arachidonic acid, which is stored in the cell membrane as esterified phospholipid until required. When macrophages are appropriately stimulated, induction of the actions of membrane-associated phospholipases occurs, and the actions catalyze the release of arachidonic acid from the phospholipids. Arahidonic acid is then oxygenated by one of two pathways. The first pathway, which is mediated by the enzyme cyclooxygenase, leads to the production of the prostaglandins (D, E, F and I series) and thromboxane (A and B series). The second pathway mediates the release of leukotrienes (A-E series) and hydroxyeicosatetraenoic acids by liposygenase. Most eicosanoids have been reported to possess immunomodulatory properties; however, the most extensively examined arachidonic metabolites with respect to effects on the immune function are probably prostaglandins.

Physiological concentrations of prostaglandin PGE_2 are important for the regulation of cyclic adenosine monophosphate (cAMP) and cyclic guanosine monophosphate (cGMP) synthesis and thereby the production of IL-2, IL-1 and TNF-α. High concentrations of PGE_2 induce the formation of cAMP which downregulate the mitogen- and antigen-activated lymphocyte proliferation, lymphocyte migration, antigen-presenting function of macrophages and the cytotoxic activity of NK cells (Fig. 10.1).[45-50]

PGE_2-inhibitors such as indomethacin enhances NK cell cytoxicity.[45-49,51,52] If the n-6/n-3 ratio on the membrane phospholipid level is shifted in favor of n-6 fatty acids this will result in an increased concentration of PGE_2 and thereby suppress the cellular immune response (Fig. 10.2). If the n-6/n-3 ratio decreases, e.g., by administration of a diet rich in n-3 fatty acids, the PGE_2-mediated immuno-suppression may be abolished (Fig. 10.2).

The interest in the role of fatty acids in the regulation of the immune response was partly stimulated by the fact that Eskimos who consumed diets relatively high in n-3 fatty acids (fish oil) had low incidences of inflammatory diseases. In autoimmune B/W female mice it was shown that n-3 dietary lipids (fish oil) increased life span, decreased autoimmunity, decreased oncogene expression (c-myc and c-Ha-ras) and increased tumor growth factor (TGF)β1. In contrast, n-6 dietary lipids (corn oil) decreased life span, accelerated the autoimmune disease progression, increased oncogene expression and decreased TGFβ1.[54] The primary effect of n-3 PUFA diet in autoimune disease is probably mediated through the reduction in prostaglandin levels with improved immune function.

In a recent review[55] on dietary fats and autoimmunity, it was concluded that the clinical benefits of n-3 fatty acids have been moderate in patients with rheumatoid arthritis. Negative results have been reported for patients with lupus nephritis, psoriasis and atopic dermatitis. Positive results have been reported for patients with Ia-nephropathy and following renal transplantation.

Increasing the concentration of n-6 PUFA in the diet have been shown to decrease T cell blastogenesis in rats, mice, rabbits and monkeys.[53] In theory, diets rich in n-6 PUFA may suppress the cellular immune response in humans. Regarding transplantation it was shown that the graft survival times of mice retreated with linoleic acid (n-6) were prolonged in comparison to those of controls or animals retreated with oleic acid.[56] This finding was evaluated in a study of 89 patients following renal transplantation

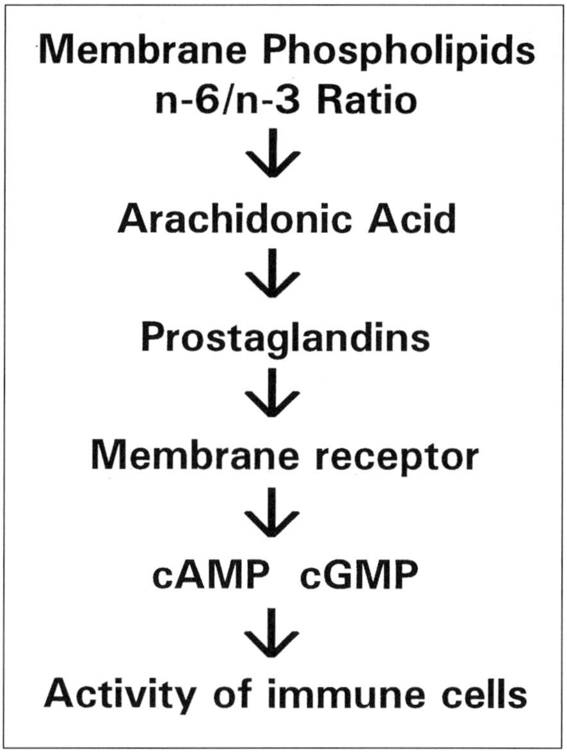

Fig. 10.1. n-6 and n-3 are precursors of eicosanoids of different series and influence thereby the function of NK and T cells.

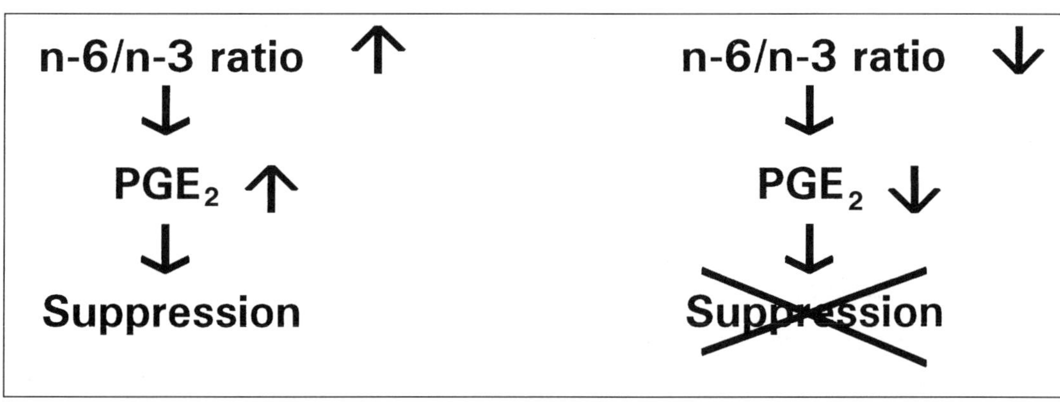

Fig. 10.2. If the n-6/n-3 ratio is shifted in favor of either n-6 or n-3 fatty acids, this will result in either increased or decreased production of PGE2. Thereby, the cellular immune system will be suppressed or the PGE2-mediated immunosuppression will be abolished.

over a follow up period of 6 months. The patients received either a diet rich in n-6 PUFA or control. The graft survival time was better in the group of patients treated with a diet high in n-6 PUFA.[57]

Little is known about the possible influence of nutritional factors on the function of NK cells. However, it was shown in a study including young healthy men that lowering the total dietary fat increased the NK activity. Furthermore, the NK cell activity returned to pre-test values when the diet was supplemented with extra fat.[59] The authors suggested that a plausible mechanism for the action of PUFA in depressing NK cell activity was related to the metabolic pathway producing 2-series prostaglandin from arachidonic acids. The relationship between PUFA in plasma and the NK cell activity was investigated in healthy elderly men.[60] A negative correlation was found between the NK cell activity and total PUFA ($r = -0.68$, $p = 0.006$), n-6 fatty acids ($r = -0.62$, $p = 0.014$) and linoleic acids ($r = -0.52$, 0.048) in plasma. In another study,[58] a negative correlation was found between linoleic acid in blood mononuclear cell (BMNC) membranes and NK cell activity ($r = -0.65$, $p = 0.01$).

Under stress conditions n-3 fatty acids may counteract latent immunosuppression by increased PGE_2 levels which appear to be further enhanced by intake of n-6 fatty acids. Under the condition of hypermetabolism, n-3 fatty acids therefore potentially act to reduce the incidence of new infections. In animal experiments, it was shown that the stress response following application of endotoxin, IL-1 or TNF was reduced when the animals were retreated with n-3 fatty acids (fish oil). The diet rich in n-3 fatty acids caused reduced catabolism, reduced febrile reaction, decreased eicosanoid production and improved survival rate.[59]

The possible interaction between intense acute exercise, known to suppress the immune system[60] and PUFA was examined in inbred female C57BI/6mice.[61] The animals received either a natural ingredient diet or a diet supplemented with various oils such as beef tallow, safflower, fish oil or linseed oil for an 8 week period. In the group receiving 18:3 (n-3) linseed oil it was shown that linseed oil abolished postexercise immunosuppression of the immunoglobulin M plaque forming cell response. Regarding the absence of exercise-induced immunosuppression in animals fed linseed oil, several mechanisms were discussed by the authors. For example, intense exercise could increase the release of catecholamines, thus increasing the catecholamine binding to adrenergic receptors. As a consequence, the stimulated protein kinase C would induce increased production of arachidonic acid and subsequently increase PGE_2 levels.

Thus, the effect of linseed oil may be ascribed to a link between a diet rich in n-3 PUFA and abolishment of prostaglandin-related immunosuppression. In support of this hypothesis, it has been shown that when the PGE_2 production was inhibited by the prostaglandin-inhibitor indomethacin, exercise-induced suppression of the NK cell activity and B cell function was partly abolished.[48,51]

NUTRITION AND AGING

Given the fact that many of the protective immune responses are impaired in old age[62,63] that nutritional deficiencies occur commonly in the elderly[64] and that nutrition is a critical determinant of immunocompetence, it has been questioned whether a causal relationship exists among nutrition, immunity and infection in old age. The pattern of illness observed in the elderly (infections, cancer and autoimmune diseases) suggests that the immune deficiency may be of clinical significance (Table 10.3).

Supplementation with selected nutrients may improve the immune system. Thus, Meydani[65] showed that both short- and longterm vitamin E supplementation enhanced the lymphocyte proliferative response, delayed type hypersensitivity and IL-2 production in healthy elderly subjects.

However, the use of a single nutrient in large doses may lead to secondary alterations in requirements, malabsorption of other nutrients and in some instances impaired immune responses. Thus excessive intake of zinc[66] or vitamins E and D[67] has been associated with impairment of the cellular immune response.

Watson et al[68] showed that supplementation with varying levels of β-carotene increased the number of $CD4^+$ cells, NK cells and IL-2 receptor expression on BMNC when the level of β–carotene supplementation was greater than 30 mg/day for 2 months. The increase in NK cells and IL-2 receptor was dose

Table 10.3. Immune alterations with aging and their sequelae

T cells	CD4/CD8↓↑ CD45RA↓ CD45R0↑ CD28↓ Proliferative response↓ DTH↓ Thymic involution
B cells	Antibody response to particular antigens↓ Autoantibodies↑ Antibody affinity↓
NK cells	Concentration/relative↑ Cytoxicity↓→
Cytokines	IL-2 production↓, IL-2R↓ IL-4 production↑↓ IFN-γ production↑↓ IL-6 production↑ TNF-α production↑
Sequelae	Incidence of infections↑ Autoimmunity↑ Cancer↑ Efficacy of vaccinations↓

dependent and the immunomodulation coincided with an increased level of plasma β-carotene but not plasma retinol.

Recently, Chandra[69] tested the hypothesis that an optimum intake of all essential micronutrients in physiological amounts would result in an improvement in immune response and reduce the frequency of infection in old age. Ninety-six healthy elderly subjects were randomly assigned to receive nutrient supplementation or placebo. The subjects were followed for 12 months. It was found that the subjects in the supplementation group had higher numbers of certain T cell subsets and NK cells, enhanced proliferative response to mitogens, increased IL-2 production, higher antibody response and increased NK activity. Furthermore, the groups receiving supplementation were less likely to have illness due to infections than those in the placebo group (23 vs. 48 days).

Regarding the immune system and lipid metabolism, indirect evidence exists that the natural immunity may be enhanced by n-3 fatty acids and suppressed by n-6 fatty acids. Several reports indicate that formation of PGE_2 increases with aging, and an increase in the sensitivity of the lymphocytes from elderly subjects to the inhibitory effects on proliferation by PGE_2 has been shown.[70]

Therefore, PGE_2-induced suppression of cell-mediated immunity by administration of n-6 fatty acids may be of special relevance to the elderly subjects and in theory, diets rich in n-3 fatty acids may enhance the immune system in elderly subjects.

EXERCISE AND AGING

As pointed out by Mazzeo,[71] it is important to know how the elderly respond and adapt to stress imposed by an acute bout of exercise. This is not only important from a mechanistic standpoint, but there are also significant clinical implications. Thus, infectious diseases are a major problem in this age group. In theory, chronic exercise training may enhance resting levels of the immune system and thus abrogate age-related immunodeficiency.

Fiatarone et al[72] examined the effect of one bout of maximal cycling in young (average age 30 years) and old (average age 71 years) women. They found no difference among the groups in the NK cell activity measured at rest or in response to acute exercise.

Crist et al[73] studied two groups of elderly women (mean = 72 years). One group participated in a program of physical training, the other group served as nonexercising controls. The resting level of NK cell activity was elevated in the trained individuals. This study thus supports the finding of increased resting levels of NK cell activity in trained versus untrained young athletes.[74,75] Interestingly, in response to acute exercise, the increase in NK cell activity in response to acute exercise was greater in trained individuals compared to untrained.[73]

Nieman et al[76] studied the basic mitogenic responses of PHA-stimulated T cells in elderly women (average age 73 years) who were in regular training for long distance running. These elite elderly subjects showed an increased proliferative response and NK cell activity compared with sedentary controls. Surprisingly, however, a 12 week training program of 30 previously sedentary women did not result in a significant increase in T cell and NK cell function despite an increase in cardiorespiratory capacity.

In a murine model, De la Fuente et al[77] measured the mitogen-induced proliferative response in spleen, thymus and axillary nodes from young and old mice. The proliferative response was lower in old mice compared to young mice. Acute exercise to exhaustion induced a decrease in mitogen-induced proliferation of both old and young untrained mice. However, chronic exercise produced an increase in the proliferative response in both old and young animals compared to sedentary animals. The acute bout of exercise was not suppressive in the trained group, and this response was found to be greater in the young compared to the old animals.

In a study by Barnes et al,[78] old Fischer rats 344 were given endurance training for a 10 week period. Old rats had a poorer antibody response than young animals; however, exercise training did not influence the antibody production to specific antigen.

Pahlavani et al[79] investigated the role of exercise training on immunosenescence in male Fischer rats 344. Rats of four different age groups were examined (1, 6, 12 and 18 months of age, initially) after a 6 month training program. An age-related decline was found in both unstimulated, mitogen-stimulated proliferation and IL-2 synthesis. It was concluded that exercise training neither prevented the age-related decline in lymphocyte proliferation nor the IL-2 production. Further, training had an adverse effect on mitogen-induced proliferation and for IL-2 production but only in the younger animals.

In another study, Nasrulla and Mazzeo[80] measured mitogen-stimulated lymphocyte proliferation, IL-2 production and NK cell cytotoxicity in splenocytes from 1, 17 and 27 month old Fischer 344 male rats. Mitogen-induced proliferation and IL-2 production were found to decrease significantly with age in both trained and untrained animals. Training significantly reduced proliferation and IL-2 production in younger animals. This is in accordance with the findings by Lin et al.[81] However, the proliferative response and the IL-2 production were found to increase in response to training in the old animals compared to the age-matched controls.

The NK cell activity declined significantly with age and training did not alter this response. The latter finding is in contrast to several other animal studies in young animals, which have shown increased resting levels of NK cell activity in response to training.[82-86]

CONCLUSION

It is not possible to conclude whether an endurance training program may alter age-related decline in immune function. The major reason for this uncertainty is related to the scarcity of data addressing the issue of exercise and immune function in elderly. There is primarily a lack of human studies. The available amount of data suggest that although age-related decline in immune function can be retarded, the greatest effect will be seen only in very highly conditioned subjects.[87]

Several studies suggest that there is a link between nutrition and immune function. Supplementation studies indicate that age-related immunodeficiency is partly due to undernutrition or malnutrition. The immunodeficiency has been shown to be partly abolished by refeeding and by small doses of vitamins. In theory, n-3 fatty acids may enhance age-related immunodeficiency and improve resistance to infections.

Few studies have addressed the potential protective role of functional food in exercise-induced immunosuppression and muscle pain. Exercise-related immunosuppression in animals was restored by a diet rich in n-3 fatty acids. Anti-oxidant supplementation has been shown to decrease the incidence of postrace URTI. Furthermore, vitamin E inhibited the acute phase response in eccentric exercise. Even though it is difficult to evaluate the individual health benefits of enhancing age- and exercise-related immunodeficiency by nutritional supplement, the total benefit to the health of the population may be substantial.

References

1. Chandra RK. Nutrition and Immunity. In: Lachmann PJ, Peters K, Rosen FS et al, eds. Clinical Aspects of Immunology. Blackwell Scientific Publications, 1993:1325-1338.
2. Chandra RK. Nutrition, immunity, and infection: present knowledge and future directions. Lancet 1983; 1(8326 Pt 1):688-691.
3. Victora CG, Barros FC, Kirkwood BR et al. Pneumonia, diarrhea, and growth in the first 4 y of life: a longitudinal study of 5914 urban Brazilian children. Am J Clin Nutr 1990; 52(2):391-396.

4. Martinez-Lopez LE, Friedl KA, Moore RJ et al. A longitudinal study of infections and injuries of Ranger students. Mil Med 1993; 158:433-437.
5. Beisel WR. History of nutritional immunology: introduction and overview. J Nutr 1992; 122(3 Suppl):591-596.
6. Gerhwin ME, Beach RS, Hurley LS. Nutrition and Immunity. New York: Academic Press, 1984:
7. Smythe PM, Brereton Stiles GG, Grace HJ et al. Thymolymphatic deficiency and depression of cell-mediated immunity in protein-calorie malnutrition. Lancet 1971; 2(731):939-943.
8. Chandra RK. Numerical and functional deficiency in T helper cells in protein energy malnutrition. Clin Exp Immunol 1983; 51(1):126-132.
9. Lesourd B. Protein undernutrition as the major cause of decreased immune function in the elderly: clinical and functional implications. Nutr Rev 1995; 53(4 Pt 2):S86-91.
10. Chandra RK. Nutrition and immunity in the elderly. Nutr Rev 1992; 50(12):367-371.
11. Hoffman-Goetz L, Keir R, Young C. Modulation of cellular immunity in malnutrition: effect of interleukin 1 on suppressor T cell activity. Clin Exp Immunol 1986; 65(2):381-386.
12. Bell RC, Hoffman-Goetz L, Keir R. Monocyte factors modulate in vitro T-lymphocyte mitogenesis in protein malnutrition. Clin Exp Immunol 1986; 63(1):194-202.
13. Chandra RK. Serum complement and immunoconglutinin in malnutrition. Arch Dis Child 1975; 50(3):225-229.
14. Haller L, Zubler RH, Lambert PH. Plasma levels of complement components and complement haemolytic activity in protein-energy malnutrition. Clin Exp Immunol 1978; 34(2):248-252.
15. Kono I, Kitao H, Matsuda M et al. Weight reduction in athletes may adversely affect the phagocytic funktions of monocytes. Phys Sportsmed 1988; 16:56.
16. Filteau SM, Menzies RA, Kaido TJ et al. Effects of exercise on immune functions of undernourished mice. Life Sci 1992; 51(8):565-74.
17. Conn CA. 13, Exercise, immunity, and dieting. In: Hoffman-Goetz L, ed. Exercise and Immune Function. New York: CRC Press, 1996:231-256.
18. Parry Billings M, Budgett R, Koutedakis Y et al. Plasma amino acid concentrations in the overtraining syndrome: possible effects on the immune system. Med Sci Sports Exerc 1992; 24 (12):1353-8.
19. Rohde T, Ullum H, Palmo J et al. Effects of glutamine on the immune system- influence of muscular exercise and HIV infection. J Appl Physiol 1995; 79(1):146-150.

20. Parry Billings M, Evans J, Calder PC et al. Does glutamine contribute to immunosuppression after major burns? Lancet 1990; 336(8714):523-525.
21. Rohde T, MacLean DA, Hartkopp A et al. The relationship between plasma glutamine level and cellular immune responses in relation to triatlon race. Eur J Appl Physiol 1996; (in press).
22. Rall LC, Meydani SN. Vitamin B6 and immune competence. Nutr Rev 1993; 51(8):217-225.
23. Beisel WR. Single nutrients and immunity. Am J Clin Nutr 1982; 35(2 Suppl):417-468.
24. Axelrod J, Trakatellis AC, Bloch H et al. Effects of pyridoxine defeciency upon delayed hypersensitivity in guinea pigs. J Nutr 1963; 79:161-167.
25. Robson LC, Schwarz MR. Vitamin B6 deficiency and the lymphoid system. II. Effects of vitamin B6 deficiency in utero on the immunological competence of the offspring. Cell Immunol 1975; 16(1):145-152.
26. Sergeev AV, Bykovskaja SN, Luchanskaja LM et al. Pyridoxine deficiency and cytotoxicity of T lymphocytes in vitro. Cell Immunol 1978; 38(1):187-192.
27. Ravn P, Linnet J, Klokker M et al. Effects of isoniazid treatment on human lymphocyte proliferative response, lymphocyte subsets and natural killer cell activity. J Immunol 1995; 30(3):247-253.
28. Chandra RK, Sudhakaran L. Regulation of immune responses by vitamin B6. Ann N Y Acad Sci 1990; 585:404-423.
29. Meydani M. Vitamin E. Lancet 1995; 345(8943):170-175.
30. Boxer LA, Oliver JM, Spielberg SP et al. Protection of granulocytes by vitamin E in glutathione synthetase deficiency. N Engl J Med 1979, 301(17):901-905.
31. Kowdley KV, Mason JB, Meydani SN et al. Vitamin E deficiency and impaired cellular immunity related to intestinal fat malabsortion. Gastroenterology 1992; 102(6):2139-2142.
32. Anderson R, Smit MJ, Joone GK et al. Vitamin C and cellular immune functions. Protection against hypochlorous acid-mediated inactivation of glyceraldehyde-3-phosphate dehydrogenase and ATP generation in human leukocytes as a possible mechanism of ascorbate-mediated immunostimulation. Ann NY Acad Sci 1990; 587:34-48.
33. Nauss KM, Phua CC, Ambrogi L et al. Immunological changes during progressive stages of vitamin A deficiency in the rat. J Nutr 1985; 115(7):909-918.
34. Friedman A, Sklan D. Antigen-specific immune response impairment in the chick as influenced by dietary vitamin A. J Nutr 1989; 119(5):790-795.

35. Peters EM, Goetzsche JM, Grobbelaar B et al. Vitamin C supplementation reduces the incidence of postrace symptoms of upper-respiratory-tract infection in ultramarathon runners. Am J Clin Nutr 1993; 57(2):170-174.
36. Peters EM, Cambell A, Pawley L. Vitamin A fails to increase resistance to upper respiratory in distance runners. S Afr J Sports Med 1992; 7:3-7.
37. Alessio HM. Exercise-induced oxidative stress. Med Sci Sports Exerc 1993; 25(2):218-224.
38. Frei B. Reactive oxygen species and antioxidant vitamins: mechanisms of action. Am J Med 1994; 97(3A):5S-13S.
39. Cannon JG, Orencole SF, Fielding RA et al. Acute phase response in exercise: interaction of age and vitamin E on neutrophils and muscle enzyme release. Am J Physiol 1990; 259(6 Pt 2): R1214-1219.
40. Cannon JG, Meydani SN, Fielding RA et al. Acute phase response in exercise. II. Associations between vitamin E, cytokines, and muscle proteolysis. Am J Physiol 1991; 260(6Pt2):R1235-1240.
41. Marshall LA, Johnston PV. The effect of dietary alpha-linolenic acid in the rat on fatty acid profiles of immunocompetent cell populations. Lipids 1983; 18(10):737-742.
42. Cleland LG, James MJ, Gibson RA et al. Effect of dietary oils on the production of n-3 and n-6 metabolites of leukocyte 5-lipoxygenase in five rat strains. Biochim Biophys Acta 1990; 1043(3):253-258.
43. Suchner U, Senftleben U. Immune modulation by polyunsaturated fatty acids during nutritional therapy: interactions with synthesis and effects of eicosanoids. Infusionsther Transfusionsmed 1994; 21(3):167-182.
44. Pruzanski W, Vadas P. Phospholipase A2—a mediator between proximal and distal effectors of inflammation. Immunol Today 1991; 12(5):143-146.
45. Brunda MJ, Herberman RB, Holden HT. Inhibition of murine natural killer cell activity by prostaglandins. J Immunol 1980; 124(6):2682-2687.
46. Droller MJ, Perlmann P, Schneider MU. Enhancement of natural and antibody-dependent lymphocyte cytotoxicity by drugs which inhibit prostaglandin production by tumor target cells. Cell Immunol 1978; 39(1):154-164.
47. Pedersen BK, Kharazmi A, Svenson M. Downregulation of natural killer cell activity by autologous polymorphonuclear leucocytes. Role of indomethacin. Allergy 1988; 43(1):17-23.
48. Pedersen BK, Tvede N, Klarlund K et al. Indomethacin in vitro and in vivo abolishes postexercise suppression of natural killer cell activity in peripheral blood. Int J Sports Med 1990; 11(2):127-131.

49. Pedersen BK, Oxholm P, Klarlund K. Characterization of the in vivo and in vitro effects of indomethacin on human natural killer cell activity. Allergy 1986; 41(7):532-536.
50. Pedersen BK, Oxholm P, Manthorpe R et al. Impaired indomethacin-boosting of the defective natural killer cell activity in patients with primary Sjogren's syndrome. Scand J Rheumatol Suppl 1986; 61:135-138.
51. Tvede N, Heilmann C, Halkjaer Kristensen J et al. Mechanisms of B-lymphocyte suppression induced by acute physical exercise. J Clin Lab Immunol 1989; 30(4):169-173.
52. Nielsen HJ, Pedersen BK, Moesgaard F et al. Effect of ranitidine on postoperative suppression of natural killer cell activity and delayed hypersensitivity. Acta Chir Scand 1989; 155(8):377-382.
53. Kelley DS, Daudu PA. Fat intake and immune response. Prog Food Nutr Sci 1993; 17(1):41-63.
54. Fernandes G, Bysani C, Venkatraman JT et al. Increased TGF-beta and decreased oncogene expression by omega-3 fatty acids in the spleen delays onset of autoimmune disease in B/W mice. J Immunol 1994; 152(12):5979-5987.
55. Endres S, De Caterina R, Schmidt EB et al. n-3 polyunsaturated fatty acids: update 1995. Eur J Clin Invest 1995; 25(9):629-638.
56. Mertin J. Effect of polyunsaturated fatty acids on skin allograft survival and primary and secondary cytotoxic response in mice. Transplantation 1976; 21(1):1-4.
57. McHugh MI, Wilkinson R, Elliot RW et al. Immunosupression with polyunsaturated fatty acids in renal transplantation. Transplantation 1977; 24:263-267.
58. Oxholm P, Pedersen BK, Horrobin DF. Natural killer cell functions are related to the cell membrane composition of essential fatty acids: differences in healthy persons and patients with primary Sjogren's syndrome. Clin Exp Rheumatol 1992; 10(3):229-234.
59. Johnson JA, 3d, Griswold JA, Muakkassa FF. Essential fatty acids influence survival in sepsis. J Trauma 1993; 35(1):128-131.
60. Hoffman-Goetz L, Pedersen BK. Exercise and the immune system: a model of the stress response? Immunol Today 1994; 15(8):382-387.
61. Benquet C, Krzystyniak K, Savard R et al. Modulation of exercise-induced immunosuppression by dietary polyunsaturated fatty acids in mice. J Tox Environm Health 1994; 43:225-237.
62. De Weck AL. Immune response and aging. In: Munro H, Schlierf G, eds. Constitutive and Environmental Aspects. New York: Raven Press, 1992:89-95.
63. Pawelec G, Adibzadeh M, Pohla H et al. Immunosenescence: ageing of the immune system. Immunol Today 1995; 16(9):420-422.

64. Chandra RK. Nutritional regulation of immunity and risk of infection in old age. Immunology 1989; 67:141-147.
65. Meydani SN. Vitamin E enhancement of T cell-mediated function in healthy elderly: mechanisms of action. Nutr Rev 1995; 53(4 Pt 2):S52-56.
66. Chandra RK. Excessive intake of zinc impairs immune responses. JAMA 1984; 252(11):1443-1446.
67. Payette H, Rola Pleszczynski M, Ghadirian P. Nutrition factors in relation to cellular and regulatory immune variables in a free-living elderly population. Am J Clin Nutr 1990; 52(5):927-932.
68. Watson R, Prabhala R, Plezia P et al. Effect of beta-carotene on lymphocyte subpopulation in elderly humans: evidene for a dose response relationship. Am J Clin Nutr 1991; 53:90-94.
69. Chandra RK. Effect of vitamin and trace-element supplementation on immune responses and infection in elderly subject. Lancet 1992; (340):1124-1127.
70. Goodwin JS, Messner RP. Sensitivity of lymphocytes to prostaglandin E2 increases in subjects over age 70. J Clin Invest 1979; 64(2):434-439.
71. Mazzeo RS. 11, Exercise, immunity, and aging. In: Hoffman-Goetz L, ed. Exercise and Immune Function. New York: CRC Press, 1996:199-214.
72. Fiatarone MA, Morley JE, Bloom ET et al. The effect of exercise on natural killer cell activity in young and old subjects. J Gerontol 1989; 44:
73. Crist DM, Mackinnon LT, Thompson RF et al. Physical Exercise Increases Natural Cellular-Mediated Tumor Cytotoxity in Elderly Women. Gerontology 1989; 35:66-71.
74. Pedersen BK, Tvede N, Christensen LD et al. Natural killer cell activity in peripheral blood of highly trained and untrained persons. Int J Sports Med 1989; 10(2):129-131.
75. Tvede N, Steensberg J, Baslund B et al. Cellular immunity in highly trained elite racing cyclists during periods of training with high and low intensity. Scand J Med Sci Sports 1991; 1:163-6.
76. Nieman DC, Henson DA, Gusewitch G et al. Physical activity and immune function in elderly women. Med Sci Sports Exerc 1993; 25(7):823-831.
77. De la Fuente M, Ferrandez MD, Miquel J et al. Changes with aging and physical exercise in ascorbic acid content and proliferative response of murine lymphocytes. Mech Ageing Dev 1992; 65(2-3):-86.
78. Barnes CA, Forster MJ, Fleshner M et al. Exercise does not modify spatial memory, brain autoimmunity, or antibody response in aged F-344 rats. Neurobiol Aging 1991; 12(1):47-53.

79. Pahlavani MA, Cheung TH, Cheskey JA et al. Influence of exercise on the immune function of rats at various ages. J Appl Physiol 1987; 1997-2001.
80. Nasrullah I, Mazzeo RS. Age-related immuno senescence in Fischer 344 rats: influence of exercise training. J Appl Physiol 1992; 73(5):1932-8.
81. Lin YS, Jan MS, Chen HI. The effect of chronic and acute exercise on immunity in rats. Int J Sports Med 1993; 14(2):86-92.
82. MacNeil B, Hoffman-Goetz L. Chronic exercise enhances in vivo and in vitro cytotoxic mechanisms of natural immunity in mice. J Appl Physiol 1993; 74(1):388-95.
83. MacNeil B, Hoffman-Goetz L. Effect of exercise on natural cytotoxicity and pulmonary tumor metastases in mice. Med Sci Sports Exerc 1993; 25(8):922-928.
84. MacNeil B, Hoffman-Goetz L. Exercise training and tumor metastasis in mice: influence of time of exercise onset. Anticancer Res 1993; 13(6A):2085-2088.
85. Hoffman-Goetz L, Arumugam Y, Sweeny L. Lymphokine activated killer cell activity following voluntary physical activity in mice. J Sports Med Phys Fit 1994; 34:83-90.
86. Hoffman-Goetz L, MacNeil B, Arumugam Y et al. Differential effects of exercise and housing condition on murine natural killer cell activity and tumor growth. Int J Sports Med 1992; 13(2):167-171.
87. Brines R, Hoffman-Goetz L, Pedersen BK. Can you exercise to make your immune system fitter? Immunol Today 1996; 17(6):252-254.

CHAPTER 11

Exercise and Cancer

Bente Klarlund Pedersen
and Inge Haunstrup Clemmensen

Physical activity is a primary strategy that has received little attention in cancer control, but an increasing number of epidemiological studies suggest a possible influence of physical activity in occupation or during leisure time on the risk of cancer.

BREAST CANCER AND CANCERS OF THE FEMALE REPRODUCTIVE SYSTEM

Breast Cancer

Breast cancer is one of the leading causes of mortality among women in the industrialized part of the world. Its incidence varies more than five-fold around the world, and the offspring of migrants moving from countries with low incidence to countries with high incidence of breast cancer acquire rates close to those of the new country, suggesting that environmental and lifestyle factors are important in the etiology of breast cancer. Even a small protective effect will have enormous influence on the cancer burden of a given population. However, although there have been several studies focusing on the primary protection against breast cancer, there have been very few positive findings. A recent report on nutrition and breast cancer[1] concludes, based on the results from large prospective studies, that there is no support for the concept developed from animals that dietary fat intake in mid-life is associated with breast cancer.

The risk factors for cancer of the breast, corpus uteri and ovary include hormonal factors. Risk factors for breast cancer include nulliparity, low parity, early menarche and late menopause.[2] To alter a woman's lifetime exposure to steroid hormones may not be feasible. However, it has been reported that premenarcheal girls who engage in strenuous physical exercise regimens may experience delay in the onset of menses.[3] Recently, a number of epidemiological studies have investigated if a relationship exists between physical activity, breast cancer and cancers of the reproductive system (Table 11.1).

The influence of occupational physical activity was investigated in three studies.[4-6] In Shanghai, Zheng et al[4] collected occupational information from 2736 women with breast cancer, 452 women with cancer of corpus uteri and 595 women with ovarian cancer. Occupational groups were classified according to job titles at time of diagnosis. Women with low activity occupations had an increased incidence of cancer of the breast, corpus uteri and ovary, whereas the incidence was reduced among women with high activity jobs when compared to the background population. However, this was only significant for breast cancer.

Vihko et al,[5] Finland, evaluated the influence of occupational physical activity by comparing two cohorts of teachers with the background population. The cancer incidence of the physical education teachers did not differ significantly from the control population, while the language teachers had a higher incidence of breast cancer compared to both the Finnish female population and the group of teachers.

In a cohort study by Vena et al[6] including 25,000 American females proportional mortality ratio was increased for breast cancer in the group with low job activity level, and decreased in the group with high job activity. Thus, the studies based on occupational physical activity[4-6] support the idea of a protective effect of physical exercise against breast cancer, or little physical activity as a risk factor for breast cancer.

Leisure time or recreational physical activity have been evaluated in several studies.[7-10] The association between recreational physical activity and breast cancer risk was examined in an

Australian population-based case control study by Friedenreich et al.[7] The women reported their level of weekly recreational physical activity in self-administered questionnaire. The questionnaire reports of light, moderate and vigorous exercise were converted into total kilocalories per week of energy expenditure. There was a trend towards a decrease in risk of breast cancer with increasing levels of total recreational physical activity.[7] Thus, the study found some evidence (of borderline statistical significance) that recreational physical activity is associated with decreased risk of breast cancer. The decrease was observed across types of recreational activity, but was most pronounced for vigorous recreational activity and was more evident in premenopausal than in postmenopausal women.

In a hospital-based case control Japanese study by Hirose et al,[8] physical activity had a protective effect against breast cancer in both pre- and postmenopausal women. This is of special interest since the etiologic factors for premenopausal breast cancer are thought to be different from those for postmenopausal breast cancer.[8] Also, the incidence rates of breast cancer in most Asian countries are much lower than those in Western countries (although there have been a marked increase in recent years).

In an American hospital-based case control study by Taiolo et al,[10] there was no association between physical activity and breast cancer. The lifetime occurrence of breast cancer and cancer of the reproductive system was determined for former college-athletes and nonathletes by Frisch et al,[9] who found an increased cancer risk for nonathletes, regarding both breast cancer and cancers of the reproductive system.

An American case control study by Bernstein et al[11] investigated young women aged 40 and younger at time for breast cancer diagnosis. This study showed that the average number of hours spent in physical activities per week was a predictor of reduced breast cancer risk.

In a recent large case control study by Mittendorf et al,[12] 6888 women with breast cancer and 9539 controls were included. In a 25 minute telephone interview information was obtained on physical activity. The study showed a 50% reduction in risk of breast cancer in those who exercised vigorously at least once a day. Among women who reported any strenuous physical activity during ages 14-22, the risk of breast cancer was reduced by 5%.

Table 11.1 Epidemiological studies on physical activity and breast cancer

Study	Site	Design Place Years of Study	Study Sample or Number of Cases	Physical Activity	Contrast	Risk
Bernstein [11] 1994	Breast	Case-control USA 1983-89	545 cases 40 years at diagnosis 545 controls	Average number of hours physical activity/week from menarche to 1 year prior to diagnosis	Inactive (ref) *vs.* $\geq$3.8 hours/ week	OR = 0.42 CI:0.27-0.64 trend P = 0.0001
Dorgan[14] 1994	Breast	Prospective cohort Framingham Heart Study 1954-56	117 cases 2,181 non-cases	Work and leisure time: hours a day spent at sleep, rest and sedentary, slight, moderate, heavy activities; converted to a physical activity index.	Quartile 1, low (ref) vs. 4	Not significant
Friedenreich[7] 1995	Breast	Population-based case-control Australia 1982-84	444 cases aged 20-74 at diagnosis 444 controls	Light, moderate, vigorous weekly recreational physical activity converted to total kilocalories/week	0 kcal/week (ref) vs. highest	Not significant
Frisch[9] 1985	Breast	Retrospective cohort USA 1925-81	2,622 college athletes 2,776 alumna=non-athletes	Athlete: at least one team for one or more years	Athletes (ref) vs. non-athletes	Not significant
Hirose[8] 1995	Breast	Hospital-based case-control Japan 1988-92	1,186 cases 607 premenopausal 445 postmenopausal 23,163 controls	Physical activity: no, occasional and > 2 times/week	No(ref) vs. > 2 times/week	OR=0.74 CI:0.55-0.99 P<0.05

Mittendorf[12] 1995	Breast	Case-control Chicago, USA 1988-91	6,888 cases 17-74 years at diagnosis 9,539 controls	Strenuous physical activity or team sports when 14-22 years of age giving a MET score	No strenuous physical activity (ref) vs. any strenuous physical activity and *vs.* at least once a day	OR = 0.95 for any CI: 0.93-0.97 OR = 0.5 at least once a day CI: 0.4-0.7
Paffenbarger[13] 1992	Breast	Cohort University of Pennsylvania, USA	2,370 alumna 25000 person-years 73 cases	Physical activity index	Less active (ref) vs. 1000 or more kcal per week	Not significant
Taioli[10] 1995	Breast	Hospital-based case-control USA 1987-90	617 cases 531 controls	Leisure time physical activity at ages 15-22 years and "any period"	No exercise (ref) vs. >20 min three times a week for 1 year or more	No significant effect and no trend
Vihko[5] 1992	Breast	Cohort Finland 1967-87	3,239 language teachers 924 physical education teachers	Language teachers and physical education teachers	Cancer incidence in the population (ref) vs. teachers	Physical education teachers:SIR=1.28 not significant. Language teachers: SIR = 1.59 p < 0.001
Vena[6] 1987	Breast	Cohort USA 1974-79	25,000 females known from death certificates	Physical activity ratings assigned to death-record occupation titles. Expected based on death rates across all jobs (excluding housewives)	Proportionate mortality ratio (PMA) = observed /expected	Activity level Low: PMA = 115 P < 0.05 High: PMA = 85 P < 0.05
Zheng[4] 1993	Breast	Record-linkage study Shanghai 1980-84	2,736 cases	Occupational physical activity. low, moderate and high converted to an energy-expenditure index	Cancer incidence in the population (ref) vs. high energy expenditure	SIR = 79 P < 0.01

OR, odds ratio; CI, confidence interval 95%; SIR, standardized incidence ratio; MET, refers to the energy expended while sitting quietly and is equivalent to 3.5 ml of oxygen per kilo of body weight per minute

In contrast to the above mentioned studies, Paffenbarger[13] found no effect of physical exercise on the incidence of breast cancer. The Framingham heart study by Dorgan et al[14] found that both moderate-to-heavy leisure and occupational activities were associated with an increased risk of breast cancer, this association was marginally significant only for leisure activity.

The epidemiological evidence concerning breast cancer in women and the protective effect of physical activity have been reviewed previously.[15-17] In line with previous reviews, we find that it is premature to make strong conclusions about the role of exercise in preventing breast cancer. However, regarding breast cancer, most studies showed either a protective effect of exercise[4-6,8,11,12] or some evidence of borderline significance,[7,9] whereas few studies have shown no significant effect and no trend[10,13] or a trend towards increased incidence of breast cancer in physically active women.[14]

Cancers of the Female Reproductive System

There are only few studies examining the association between exercise and endometria cancer or other cancers of the reproductive tract. However, exercise does not seem to play an important protective role. Although one study showed that high versus low physical activity measured as house work protected against endometria cancer,[18] and another study found that there was an increased risk for cancers of the reproductive system (uterus, cervix, ovary and vagina) for nonathletes compared with former college-athletes,[9] other studies have not found any significant influence of physical activity on endometria cancer.[4,19,20]

Possible Mechanisms

The role of endogenous estrogens in the development of breast cancer has been under extensive scientific interest. Strenuous physical exercise decreases the estrogen level and is associated with delay in the onset of menses, and an increase in the number of anovulatory cycles. Exercise may ultimately alter the lifetime exposure to estrogens.

It is not known if natural immune changes associated with exercise and training may have biological relevance for the development of breast cancer. It has been shown that exogenous β-estradiol increases tumor metastasis and natural immune suppression in mice. Adoptive transfer of normal spleen cells enhanced the NK cell activity and increased the resistance of estradiol-treated mice to tumor metastasis.[21]

In an experimental study by Hoffman-Goetz et al,[22] it was examined whether exercise influenced the experimental metastasis of a mouse mammary tumor. After 8 weeks of forced treadmill exercise or voluntary wheel running, female BALB/c mice received an intravenous injection of MMT line 66 tumor cells. Mice were then randomized into continuation of activity, cessation of activity, initiation of activity and maintenance of sedentary condition for 3 weeks. The lymphokine activated killer (LAK) cell activity measured in vitro was enhanced in the trained, compared to the sedentary, animals. However, endurance training did not alter the development of tumor metastasis.

The MMT66 is a highly aggressive tumor cell line that is only partially LAK sensitive, and since interleukin (IL)-2 was not administered in vivo the lack of significance was not surprising. Interestingly, it was found that tumor multiplicity was lower in animals trained (and then rested) prior to tumor inoculation than in animals that either continued exercise during tumor metastasis or that were sedentary throughout the study.[17,22]

In two other studies by MacNeil and Hoffman-Goetz,[23,24] trained mice had higher in vitro natural killer (NK) cell activity, greater lung clearance of radiolabeled CIRAS tumor cells and lower absolute tumor incidence.

Woods et al[25,26] found that exercise enhanced in vitro macrophage antitumor cytotoxicity, but that the number of metastases of a mouse mammary adenocarcinoma did not differ between control mice that were exercised 3 days before tumor injection and 14 days after.[27]

In a recent review by Hoffman-Goetz and Husted,[17] it is concluded that for tumors that are insensitive to natural immune control, and for those that are highly aggressive, exercise may have little or even negative consequences. Thus, the underlying mechanisms regarding influence of exercise training on breast cancer are likely to include tumor characteristics, host characteristics, exercise characteristics and timing of exercise.

CANCERS OF THE MALE REPRODUCTIVE SYSTEM

PROSTATE CANCER

Prostate cancer is a common cancer in many Western countries although it is relatively rare among Asian men. Despite its high incidence in Western countries, little is known about prostate cancer etiology. However, production or metabolism of androgenic hormones have been proposed in the development of prostate cancer.[28,29]

Physical activity may induce lower circulating levels of testosterone.[30-32] Therefore, an active and fit way of life may in theory prevent or delay the clinical progression of prostate cancer. The international and interethnic differences in prostate cancer incidence also suggest that environmental factors may be of importance. A number of epidemiological studies on exercise, prostate and testicular cancers have been performed (Table 11.2).

Vena et al[33] reported in a cohort study evaluating the influence of occupation titles that the proportionate mortality ratio = observed/expected death cases from prostate cancer was lower in active individuals and higher in individuals with sedentary jobs. In a study from Hawaii, Marchand et al[34] also found in men older than 70 years a negative association between prostate cancer risk and proportion of life spent in jobs involving only sedentary or light work. The negative association was dependent on amount of work, consistent across ethnic groups, and unrelated to socioeconomic status, dietary risk factors or job-related chemical exposures. However, the findings in younger men were less clear, but not inconsistent with those for older men.

In a case cohort study, Hsing et al[35] found a small excess risk of borderline significance of prostate cancer among white-collar workers and occupations with low physical activity levels in urban Shanghai, an area where prostate cancer is relatively rare and physical activity relatively high.

The effect of self-reported occupational physical activity on prostate cancer was evaluated by Whittemore et al.[36] In this study four ethnic groups were included (black, white; Chinese-American and Japanese-American). The study found no consistent associations between prostate cancer risk and any measure of physical activity.

In the study by Paffenbarger et al,[13] physical activity level was assessed in 1962 or 1966 and in 1977 among college alumni. As in the study of colon cancer, they found that active alumni had the same risk of developing prostate cancer as their inactive counterparts when a single assessment of physical activity was made. However, when activity was jointly assessed in 1962, 1966 and 1977 the findings were different for older alumni. Similar results were later reported by the same authors.[37]

In two case control studies, Yu et al,[38] USA, and Andersson et al,[39] Sweden, found borderline significant effects of physical exercise on prostate cancer during adulthood[38] and childhood,[39] respectively.

Regarding prostate cancer, most studies have shown either a protective effect of exercise[13,33,34] or some evidence of borderline significance,[35,38,39] whereas one study showed no effect and no trend.[36] No studies found a positive association between prostate cancer and physical activity. However, it is still premature to conclude that exercise protects against the development of prostate cancer.

Testis Cancer

Testicular cancer has increased markedly in young white populations throughout the past 20-40 years and is in many Western countries the most common form of cancer in men aged 20-34 years. Apart from a history of undescended testis no risk factors have been identified with certainty. Sharpe and Skakkebœk[40] have proposed that a common factor, exposure to environmental oestrogens in utero, may be responsible for both a reported decreased sperm count and an increased risk of testicular cancer in developed countries.

A model has also been proposed of the development of testicular cancer[41] based on increased exposure to pituitary gonadotropin. These hormones may increase the rates of germ cell mitosis and thereby influence tumor development. The model is clearly speculative. However, in theory environmental factors such as exercise may influence the hormone profile and thereby the development of testicular cancer.

A large interview-based case control study was performed by the United Kingdom testicular cancer study group.[41] The risk of

Table 11.2. ***Epidemiological studies on physical activity, prostate and testicular cancers***

Study	Site	Design, Place, Years of Study	Study Sample/ Number of Cases	Physical Activity	Contrast	Risk
Andersson[39] 1995	Prostate	Case-control Sweden 1989-92	256 cases and 252 controls	Level of physical activity during puberty.	Comparison with classmates (lower, same, higher).	Not significant.
Gallagher[42] 1995	Testis	Case-control Canada 1980-85	510 cases aged 15-79 996 controls	Mean annual metabolic-weighted sport score all ages. Job score from age 20. Quartiled.	1) Recreational activity level lowest (ref) *vs.* rest. 2) Occupational activity level 1 (ref) *vs.* rest.	1) OR = 0.7 CI: 0.5-0.9 P trend = 0.003. 2) not significant.
Hsing[35] 1994	Prostate	Case-cohort Shanghai 1980-84	264 cases	Occupational data from the 1982 census and interviews from retired, grouped into low-, moderate- and high-activity groups.	SIR (observed to expected for urban Shanghai). Observed in three groups: low (<8 kj/min), moderate (8-12 kj/min), high (>12 kj/min).	Not significant
Lee[37] 1992	Prostate	Cohort USA 1965-77 and 1980-88	17719 Harvard alumni 419 prostate cases	Self-reported physical activity assessed twice (stair climbing, walking, sports).	Inactive in both 1962/66 and 1977 (ref) *vs.* highly active in both 1962/66 and 1977.	RR = 0.12 CI:0.02-0.89.
Le Marchandet[34] 1991	Prostate	Population-based case-control Hawaii 1977-83	452 cases and 899 controls	Lifetime occupational history. Jobtitle assigned one of five levels and proportion of work years in these levels.	Proportion of total life in jobs with sedentary or light work 0.00 (ref) *vs.* >0.54 for men aged $\geq$ 70.	OR = 0.5 CI: 0.3-0.9.

Paffenbarger[13] 1992	Prostate	Cohort USA 1966-77 and 1977-88	Harvard College 419 cases aged 30-79 228,000 person-years	Physical activity levels assessed 1962/66 and 1977.	Physically inactive at both questionnaire (ref) *vs.* active both years.	RR = 0.53 CI: 0.29-0.95 only for men aged ≥70 expending more 4000 kcal per week, no dose-response relationship. Other results not significant.
Thune[43] 1994	Prostate and testis	Population-based cohort Norway 1972-78	53,242 men aged 19-50	Self-reported recreational and occupational physical activity graded 1-4.	Occupational sedentary (ref) *vs.* occ. heavy and recreational sedentary (ref) *vs.* regularly training.	Not significant.
United Kingdom Testicular Cancer Study Group[41] 1994	Testis	Population-based case-control United Kingdom 1984-87	794 cases aged 15-49 609 controls	1) Hours of exercise a week at reference age. 2) Hours spent sitting down a day at reference day.	1) None (ref) *vs.* >15. 2) 0-2 (ref) *vs.* >10.	1) OR = 0.62 CI: 0.42-0.91 trend P = 0.010. 2) OR = 1.71 CI: 1.08-2.72 trend P = 0.006.
Whittemore[36] 1995	Prostate	Case-control USA and Canada 1989-91	1,655 cases (black, white, Chinese-American, Japanese-American) and 1,645 controls	Occupational self-reported on-the-job physical activity in 3 categories. Light and moderate activity for a typical 24-hours day.		No consistent associations between cancer risk and any measure of physical activity.
Vena[33] 1987	Prostate	Cohort New York 1950-79	430,000 males known from death certificates	Physical activity ratings assigned to death-record occupation titles. Expected based on death rates across all jobs.	Proportionate mortality ratio = observed/expected.	Activity level Low: PMA = 109 $P < 0.05$. High: PMA = 93 $P < 0.05$.
Yu[38] 1988	Prostate	Case-control New York 1969-84	1,162 cases and 3,124 controls	Physical exercise during adulthood, three groups.	Active (ref) *vs.* seldom.	$OR_{whites} = 1.3$ CI = 1.0- 1.6 trend P = 0.03

OR, odds ratio; CI, confidence interval 95%; RR, relative risk; PMR, proportionate mortality ratio testicular cancer decreased with increased amount of exercise and increased with increased sedentary time. The study confirmed previous findings in a case control study by Gallagher et al,[42] Canada, showing that a moderate to high level of recreational activity level was associated inversely with testicular cancer risk. When periods of life were examined, similar associations were seen with physical activity level during childhood, adolescence and adulthood. However, the strongest trend in decreased risk was seen with lifetime mean, annual recreational level. This may suggest that continuing with a modest level of activity may have the strongest effect on overall risk of testicular cancer.[42]

Thus, two studies on testis cancer showed a protective effect of physical activity on testis cancer,[41,42] but a population-based cohort study by Thune et al,[43] Norway, found no association between physical activity and testicular cancer. Clearly, the number of studies are too few and does not allow to draw any conclusions on exercise and testis cancer.

Possible Mechanisms

Several hypotheses exist regarding the influence of hormonal factors (estrogens, androgens, gonadotropin) on the development of prostate and testicular cancers. Exercise plays a potential role in modulating the hormone profiles, but given the lack of empirical data in this area, it is not possible to suggest mechanisms of action for exercise, hormone production and cancer. Furthermore, there are no evidence for a role of the immune system in linking exercise and cancers of the male reproductive tract.

COLON AND RECTAL CANCER

Colorectal cancer is one of the most common cancers in developed societies.[44] Considerable efforts have focused on identifying lifestyle-related factors to reduce the morbidity- and mortality-associated with the colorectal cancer. However, most studies have focused on dietary factors. That physical activity may reduce the risk of colon cancer was suggested already in 1981 by Persky et al[45] who found an association between heart rate and colon cancer.

In reviewing the epidemiological literature (Table 11.3) with respect to colorectal cancer, it is important to distinguish between colon and rectal cancer, since results on risk factors have not been consistent between the two sites.

In 1984, Garabrant et al[46] reported a study on 2950 population-based colon cancer cases in American males. To determine if colon cancer risk was reduced by physical activity on the job in males, the authors first rated each occupation by judging the activity level as high, moderate or sedentary. Men with sedentary jobs had a colon cancer risk at least 1.6 times that of men whose jobs required a high level of activity. Risk increased in a stepwise manner as activity level decreased.

In 1985, Vena et al[47] showed in a case control study that risk of colon cancer increased as years spent in jobs with sedentary or light work increased. Lifetime occupational history was evaluated by job title coded into five categories of physical activity. Persons who spent all their work years in jobs with sedentary or light work had twice the risk for colon cancer as compared with those never employed in jobs with sedentary or light work. A dose-response relationship was seen, with increasing risk associated with an increasing proportion of years in jobs with sedentary or light work.

Since the original observations by Garabrant et al[46] and Vena et al,[47] several studies from many countries have investigated the influence of occupational activity on the incidence of colon cancer.[48-68]

A cohort study by Fraser and Pearce,[48] New Zealand, showed that relative to males in high physical activity occupation, males in sedentary occupations had an increased incidence of both cancer of the colon and rectum.

Occupational data from patients with colon cancer were compared to the background population in a study by Chow et al,[49] Shanghai. Men employed in occupations with low physical activity levels had modest but significant elevated risks of colon cancer.

In a population-based case control study by Whittemore et al[50] on colorectal cancer among Chinese men and women in Western North America and the People's Republic of China, it was found that colon cancer was increased among men employed in sedentary occupations. On both continents and in both sexes, risk for colon cancer increased with increasing time spent by sitting. Among immigrants to North America, the risk increased with increasing numbers of years lived in North America. It was suggested that

Table 11.3. Epidemiological studies on physical activity, colon and rectal cancers

Study	Site	Design Place Years of study	Study Sample or Number of Cases	Physical Activity	Contrast	Risk
Arbman[59] 1993	Colon and rectum	Case-control Sweden 1984-86	98 colon 79 rectal 801 controls	Three levels of occupational physical activity. Employment years	Sedentary work: 0 year (ref) *vs.* >20 year	Rectal OR = 0.3 CI: 0.1-0.8 Not significant for active work and not significant for colon.
Ballard-Barbash[74] 1990	Colon	Population-based prospective cohort The Framingham Study 1954-82	1,906 men 73 cases 2,308 women 79 cases	Summary of time spent per 24 hours calculated to a physical activity index	Highest tertile (34-83) (ref) *vs.* middle and lowest tertiles	Not significant
Brownson[68] 1989	Colon	Case-control Missouri, Columbia 1984-87	1,993 cases 9,965 controls men	Three levels of occupational physical activity	High (ref) *vs.* low	OR = 1.4 CI:1.0-1.9 trend 0.02NBNBNB not significant
Chow[49] 1993	Colon	Record-linkage study Shanghai 1980-84	2,000 cases resident of Shanghai >30 years of age	Low, medium and high occupational physical activity converted to an energy-expenditure index	Cancer incidence in the population (ref) *vs.* high energy expenditure	SIR = 85 men CI: 74-97 P trend < 0.01 SIR = 83 women CI: 67-101 P trend < 0.01
Fraser & Pearce[48] 1993	Colon and rectum	Cohort New Zealand 1972-80	1651 colon cases 1046 rectum cases men aged 15-64	Current occupation classified as sedentary, intermediate or high physical activity	High (ref) *vs.* sedentary	Colon: RR = 1.18 CI: 1.02-1.36 Rrectum: RR = 1.26 CI: 1.04-1.52
Fredriksson[60] 1989	Colon	Case-control Umeå, Sweden 1980-83	329 cases 658 controls men and women aged 30-75	3 levels of occupational physical activity; employment years	Low (ref) *vs.* high	OR = 0.82 men chi-square value 27.3 OR = 0.68 women chi-square value 141.4

Garabrant[46] 1984	Colon and rectum	Cohort California, USA 1972-81	2950 cases men aged 20-64	Occupation leveled high, moderate or sedentary	High (ref) *vs.* sedentary	RR = 1.6 CI:1.3-1.8 Rectum not significant
Gerhardsson[51] 1986	Colon and Rectum	Cohort Sweden 1961-79	7115 colon 5290 rectum all working men aged 20-64 born in Sweden	Physical job activity converted to sitting time during working hours	Physically active jobs (ref) *vs.* sedentary jobs	Colon RR = 1.3 CI 90%: 1.2-1.5 Rectum not elevated
Gerhardsson[53] 1988	Colon	Cohort Sweden 1969-82	16477 twins	Questionnaire on occupational and recreational physical activity	Regular and hard exercise and physical demanding (ref) *vs.* sedentary	RR = 3.6 CI: 1.3-9.8
Gerhardsson[63] 1990	Colon and rectum	Population-based case-referent Stockholm, Sweden 1986-88	452 colon 268 rectum 624 referents	3 levels of physical activity, working hours and recreational hours every 5 years 1950-85	Very active (ref) *vs.* sedentary	Not significant
Giovannucci[70] 1995	Colon	Prospective cohort study Massachusetts 1986-92	47,723 health professionals aged 40-75	Leisure time physical activity converted to an energy expenditure index (MET-hours)	0.9 MET-hours (ref) *vs.* 46.8 MET- hours	RR = 0.53 CI:0.32-0.88 trend P=0.03
Jarebinski[64] 1988	Colon and rectum	Case-control Yugoslavia 1984-86	186 colon and rectum 372 controls	Job activity	Active (ref) *vs.* sedentary	Not significant
Kotake[66] 1995	Colon and rectum	Case-control Japan 1992-94	363 cases 363 controls	Self estimates on physical activity categorized as sedentary, fairly active and very active	Very active (ref) *vs.* sedentary	Not significant
Kune[55] 1990	Colon and rectum	Case-control study Australia 1980-81	388 male cases and 398 controls 327 females cases and 329 controls	Occupational, home and other recreational activities. All activities levels in 5 groups	Not very active retired or in verysedentary occupations (ref) *vs.* busy housewives/active retired or *vs.* moderate and strenuous activity	Not significant

continued...

Table 11.3. Epidemiological studies on physical activity, colon and rectal cancers (continued)

Study	Site	Design Place Years of study	Study Sample or Number of Cases	Physical Activity	Contrast	Risk
Lee[72] 1991	Colon and rectum	Prospective cohort USA 1962-88	225 colon 44 rectum 20775 alumni	Two assessments: 1962/66 and 1977, climbing, walking, sport converted to energy expenditure index	Inactive (ref) vs. moderately active (both in 1962/66 and in 1977)	RR: 0.52 CI:0.28-0.94 Rectum not significant
Lee & Paffenbarger[73] 1994	Colon and rectum	Cohort Harvard Alumni Health Study 1962-88	17,607 men aged 30-79 year 244 colon 53 rectal	Selfreported physical activity twice (1962/ and 1977) converted to an energy-expenditure index	Inactive (ref) vs. highly active	Not significant
Longnecker[61] 1995	Right colon & rectum	Case-control USA 1986-88	163 colon 242 rectum 242 rectum 703 controls men only	Occupation given a physical activity score:sedentary, light, moderate, heavy leisure time: 0, <.5, 1 or 2 hours per weekper week	Occ: sedentary (ref) *vs.* light, moderate, heavy No exercise (ref) *vs.* >2 hours	Not significant
Marcus[75] 1994	Colon	Case-control Wisconsin 1990-91	536 cases 2,315 controls women, less than 75 year	Strenuous activity during ages 14-22	No activity (ref) *vs.* any activity	Not significant
Markowitz[54] 1992	Colon and rectum	Case-control USA 1985	90,440 cases men 1,164 controls	Recreational activity >20 min 3 x week for >1year Occupational activity high, moderate and low activity	Low (ref) *vs.* high occupational activity	Colon OR = 0.5 CI: 0.3-0.8 Rectum not significant
Paffenbarger[13] 1992	Colon	Cohort Harvard College, USA 1966-77 and 1977-88	72,000 person-years 110 cases	Physical activity levels assessed 1962/66 and 1977	Physically inactive at both questionnaire (ref) *vs.* active both years	RR = 0.52 90% CI: 0.28- 0.94
Peters[58] 1989	Colon and rectum	Case-control study California 1974-82	147 men under 45 years of age at diagnose with colorectal cancer	Estimated activity and hours spent active from job title, and summing four cross-product terms	Moderately active (ref) vs. mainly sedentary	Transverse/ descending colon OR = 3.0 CI: 1.2-7.2 All other results not significant

Severson[69] 1989	Colon and rectum	Cohort Hawaii 1965-68, follow-up to 1986	8,006 Japanese men on Hawaii	Summary weighted physical activity index based on appr. oxygen consumption spent per 24 hours. Subjects semiquantative estimates of the amount of physical activity on the job and at home /recreation	1) physical activity index tertile 1st = 0-30.1 (ref) *vs.* 2nd = 30.2-34.2 2) physical activity at home: mostly sitting (ref) *vs.* moderate or heavy	1) colon: RR = 0.56 CI:0.39-0.80 Other sites not significant 2) colon: RR = 0.66 CI:0.49-0.88 Other sites not significant
Slattery[57] 1988	Colon	Case-control Utah 1979-83	119 female cases 204 controls 110 male cases and 180 male controls	Leisure time Occupational activity converted to an energy-expenditure index	MALES: intense activity none (ref) *vs.* high FEMALES: total activity low (ref) *vs.* high	OR = 0.29 (males) 90% CI: 0.12-0.69 OR= 0.51 (females) 90% CI: 0.29-0.91
Slattery[56] 1990	Colon	Case-control Utah, USA 1979-81	231 cases 391 controls	5 levels of physical job activity using the Dictionary of Occupational Titles and self-reported amount of time spent in light, moderate and intense types of leisure time activity and occupational activity	Total self-reported low (ref) *vs.* high	Women OR = 0.5 90% CI: 0.3-0.9 All other results not significant
Thun[65] 1992		Prospective case-control USA 1982-88	764,343 adults 1150 deaths from colon cancer 5746 controls	Physical activity in work or play (none, slight, moderate, heavy)	None (ref) *vs.* slight, moderate, heavy	Not significant
Vena[47] 1985	Colon and rectum	Case-control Buffalo, New York 1957-65	210 colon 276 rectum 1,431 controls aged 30-79 males only	Lifetime occupational history, jobtitle coded into five categories of physical activity	No. of years in jobs with sedentary/light work: none (ref) vs. > 20	Colon OR = 2.05 $p < 0.001$ No association for rectum

continued...

Table 11.3. Epidemiological studies on physical activity, colon and rectal cancers (continued)

Study	Site	Design Place Years of study	Study Sample or Number of Cases	Physical Activity	Contrast	Risk
Vena[6] 1987	Colon and rectum	Cohort USA 1950-79	430,000 males known from death certificates	Known from death certificates: physical activity ratings assigned to death-record occupation titles and expected deaths from cancers was based on proportionate death rates across all jobs	PMA = proportionate mortality ratio = observed/expected	Activity level Colon Low: PMA = 120 $P < 0.01$ High: PMA = 89 $P < 0.01$ Rectum Low: PMA = 116 $P < 0.01$ High: PMA = 89 $P < 0.05$
Vetter[62] 1992	Colon	Case-control Turkey 1979-84	107 cases 486 controls	Occupational physical activity spent sitting, and energy expenditure-time	High (ref) vs. mod. and sed.	Not significant
Vineis[67] 1993	Colon	Hospital case-referent Torino 1989-91	131 cases 463 controls	All jobs classified to energy expenditure	>12 kj/min (ref) vs. less than 8 kj/min	Not significant
Whittemore[50] 1990	Colon and rectum	Population based case-control North America and China 1981-86	905 cases 2,488 controls	Occupational and leisure time activity converted to daily energy output	Active (ref) *vs.* sedentary lifestyle	USA colon OR = 1.6 men CI:1.1-2.4 OR = 2.0 women CI: 1.2-3.3 Rectum not significant China not significant
Wu[71] 1987	Colorectal	Prospective cohort California 1981-85	11,644 residents in a retirement community: 58 male and 68 female incident colorectal cancers	Time per day spent in physical activities physical activity	<1 hr/day (ref) *vs.* >2 hr/day	Males: 0.40 CI: 0.2-0.8 Females not significant

colon cancer risk increased with duration of exposure to a sedentary lifestyle and to a diet rich in saturated fat.

The association between physical job activity and colon cancer was examined in a 19 year followup study of 1.2 million Swedish men in a study by Gerhardsson.[51] The relative risk of colon cancer in men employed in sedentary occupations was increased, while the relative risk for rectal cancer was not elevated. The same results were found in a Danish cohort study by Lynge et al.[52] In a 14 year followup on the Swedish population-based study by Gerhardsson et al,[53] a 3-fold increase in colon cancer was found among subjects with low physical activity.

Five case control studies from North America by Markowitz et al,[54] Slattery et al,[56,57] Peters et al[58] and two studies from Sweden by Arbman et al[59] and Fredriksson et al[60] showed that occupational activity was protective with respect to colon cancer irrespective of whether one engaged in recreational activity at any different period of life.[54] The same trend (not significant) was found in another American case control study by Longnecker et al,[61] in studies by Brownson et al,[68] Columbia, Vetter et al,[62] Turkey, Gerhardsson et al,[63] Sweden, Jarebinski et al,[64] ex-Yugoslavia, and by Fredriksson et al,[60] Japan.

An American prospective case control study by Thun et al[65] based on mortality, a study by Kotake et al,[66] Japan and a study by Vineis,[67] Italy, failed to show any association between occupational activity and colon cancer. Furthermore, in an Australian case control study by Kune et al[55] there was no association between colorectal cancer and physical activity. In the latter study[55] the authors did not separate colon and rectum cancer, and there were relatively few individuals with high level of physical activity.

Most epidemiological studies have measured physical activity indirectly, thus occupation has been used as a surrogate measure of physical activity. However, in a prospective study by Severson et al,[69] a summary of physical activity index measuring both occupational and leisure activities was calculated. There was a strong inverse association between the level of physical activity (estimated by the activity index and resting heart rate) and colon cancer.

The influence of leisure activity on colon cancer based on questionnaires have been studied in a number of studies.[70-74] An American cohort study by Giovannucci et al[70] evaluated leisure physical activity converted to an energy expenditure index and showed an inverse association between physical activity and risk for colon cancer. Similar results were obtained in another American prospective cohort study by Wu et al.[71] The results were consistent for both men and women, but the finding was only significant for men.[71]

In a third American cohort study, Lee et al[72] evaluated physical activity in college alumni based on self-report stair climbing, walking and sports play assessed at two time points (1962, 1966 and 1977). Alumni who were highly active at both assessments had half the risk of developing colon cancer relative to those who were inactive at both assessments. Using both assessments concurrently may have allowed alumni who were "truly" active to be correctly separated from those truly inactive. The same trend (same study?) was presented later.[73]

In a retrospective case control study by Markus et al[75] there was no significant association between strenuous physical activity during ages 14-22 and colon cancer in a group of Wisconsin women. However, the odds ratio for daily activity were below 0.50, but they were not significant and were based on very few women. In the Framingham study by Ballard-Barbas,[74] inactivity was associated with an increased risk of large bowel cancer in men (only significant at low BMI) but not in women.

The epidemiological data on colon cancer and exercise is remarkable consistent as recently pointed out by Hoffman-Goetz and Husted[76] and as suggested previously by Macfarlane and Lowenfels.[77] Despite the fact that different methods of assessing the amount of physical exercise of individuals were applied and that different types of physical activity were measured, there is consistent evidence that people with sedentary jobs, decreased participation in leisure or recreational activities, or minimal total physical activity have an increased risk of colon cancer. There is no evidence for a role of exercise in rectal cancer.

Possible Mechanisms

The potential mechanisms through which exercise may confer a protective effect against colon cancer have recently been reviewed.[17,76] These mechanisms include exercise-associated changes in gut peristalsis, and concentration of fecal bile acids in stool,[78] whereas the mechanisms seem to be largely independent of the cellular immune system. However, Hoffman-Goetz and Husted[76] recently suggested that cytokines may play a pathogenetic role in the development of colon cancer.[76]

The ability to generate IL-1 was studied in W/Fu rats bearing syngenic colon carcinomas. During local tumor growth there was a decrease in the capacity of the mononuclear cells of the host to generate IL-1. The presence of large tumor burden or metastases resulted in a further sharp fall in IL-1 generation.[79] Others have described that IL-1 release by mononuclear cells stimulated with lipopolysaccharide is decreased in many cancer patients.[80]

Eccentric exercise associated with muscle damage has been shown to enhance the circulating levels of inflammatory cytokines, including IL-1, IL-6 and tumor necrosis factor (TNF)-α.[81-88] The in vitro production of IL-1 and IL-6 was enhanced following acute concentric exercise.[89] In line with the hypothesis that high levels of IL-1 could stimulate adhesion of tumor cells to extracellular matrix and provide opportunities for innate immune responses such as surface phagocytosis or increased NK cell recycling for tumor target, exercise-mediated increase in IL-1 might be expected to reduce tumor metastasis.

OTHER CANCERS

The causes of renal cell cancer, which is relatively common in many Western countries, with high incidence rates particularly in Scandinavia[90] are poorly understood. Besides smoking, obesity remains the only risk factor that is fairly well-established.[91-94] The association between weight or body mass index have been more consistent for women than for men, and some evidence exists for an influence of weight cycling in women.[91] Furthermore, an association with reproductive variables, including decreased risk for women with late menarche and first pregnancy and birth have been suggested.[93] A handful of studies[91-94] have evaluated the effect of physical activity (leisure and working) on renal cell cancer and found no influence of physical exercise.

In a cohort study from Great Britain by Stukonis and Doll[95] the mortality rate showed a marked trend with physical activity. It was suggested that the positive relationship between the mortality from gastric cancer and physical activity at work was partly due to the fact that men whose occupation involves heavy work eat more and are consequently exposed to a greater quantity of carcinogens in their food. Premature results from the Japan-Hawaii Cancer Study by Severson et al[69] supported this finding. However, a later report on the same cohort concluded that there was no significant influence of physical activity.[96]

A number of studies have evaluated the influence of physical activity of all cancers[97-104] or many cancers,[105,106] but the results have been very inconsistent showing both positive and negative associations.

CONCLUSION

There is substantial evidence accumulating for a protective role of exercise in colon cancer risk. Although there is the same trend in breast cancer and prostate cancer, it is premature to draw strong conclusions regarding a potential effect of exercise. The role of exercise in tumorigenesis is probably based on multiple and overlapping mechanisms of action. These include altered peristalsis, bile acid composition, diets, prostaglandins and cytokines. Exercise is known to induce dramatic changes in hormonal factors and may thereby exert its effect on tumor growth. The exercise-induced effect on sex hormones may directly influence the tumor growth of some cancers such as breast cancer and prostate cancer. However, experimental evidence also suggest that estrogens may influence tumor growth by natural immune suppression.[21] Certainly, exercise induces dramatic changes in neuroendocrine factors, which again cause alterations in the cellular immune system, especially in natural immunity.[107] There is, however, a clear need for well-designed investigations to address the putative interactions among exercise, natural immunity and cancer. A common assumption is that because chronic training enhances natural immunity, enhanced natural immunity could reduce tumor growth. This approach has, however, not been experimentally invalidated. One study showed that pretreatment of mice with an antibody against NK cells (anti-asialo-GM1) completely abolished the exercise effects on in vitro cytotoxicity and partially abrogated the in vivo cytotoxicity effect as well as the tumor count.[24] Although these findings suggest a link between exercise training and reduced metastasis mediated through natural immune factors, this interpretation is strongly influenced by the specific tumor model used, exercise characteristics and timing of exercise.

The theory that cancer may arise in a host under conditions of reduced immune capacity was first put forward by Thomas[108] in 1959, and later developed in the theory of immune surveillance by Burnet[109] in 1965.

Although this hypothesis in its original form has been abandoned, the role of the immune system in the neoplastic process was supported by observations in experimental animals.[110] More recent animal data, however, have indicated that the immune system is involved primarily in malignancies of viral origin.[111]

This is in accordance with the finding of increased incidence of specific cancers in patients with acquired immunodeficiency syndrome (AIDS). These cancers are non-Hodgkins lymphoma, Kaposi's sarcoma, anal cancer and cervical cancer, which have all been shown to be of viral origin.[112] Nevertheless, reports of patients with immune impairment caused by immunosuppressive treatment, as seen after kidney transplantation, show an excess of cancer where a viral etiology is not known.[113] However, there are no reasons to believe that the list of cancers caused by an infection is now complete. In recent years, microorganisms have been linked to a couple of new cancers. Thus, herpes virus type 8 has been identified as the cause of Kaposis sarcoma[114] and gastric infection with *Helicobacter pylori* has been identified as a risk factor for gastric cancer.[115]

Regarding the acute exercise effects on the immune response, it has been shown that natural immunity is enhanced during moderate and severe exercise. However, the numbers and function of cells mediating cytotoxic activity against virus-infected and tumor target cells are suppressed after intense, long-term exercise.[107,116-118]

In accordance with the immune surveillance theory, it was therefore to be expected that moderate exercise protected against malignancy whereas exhaustive exercise was linked with increased cancer risk. Today there are limited data to support this theory. Although the majority of epidemiological studies show that physical activity as such protects against cancer, there is until now, only one study on subjects who have performed extreme amounts of strenuous exercise for a long period of their life. The latter study showed increased cancer risk in association with exhaustive training and thus found some evidence of support for the immune surveillance theory.[119]

References

1. Hunter DJ, Willett WC. Nutrition and breast cancer. Cancer Causes Control 1996; 7:56-68.
2. Kelsey JL, Gammon MD. The epidemiology of breast cancer. Cancer J Clin 1991; 41:146-165.
3. Warren MP. The effects of exercise on pubertal progression and reproductive function in girls. J Clin Endocrinol Metab 1980; 51:1150-1157.
4. Zheng W, Shu XO, McLaughlin JK et al. Occupational physical activity and the incidence of cancer of the breast, corpus uteri, and ovary in Shanghai. Cancer 1993; 71:3620-3624.
5. Vihko VJ, Apter DL, Pukkala EI et al. Risk of breast cancer among female teachers of physical education and languages. Acta Oncol 1992; 31:201-204.
6. Vena JE, Graham S, Zielezny M et al. Occupational exercise and risk of cancer. Am J Clin Nutr 1987; 45:318-327.
7. Friedenreich CM, Rohan TE. Physical activity and risk of breast cancer. Eur J Cancer Prev 1995; 4:145-151.
8. Hirose K, Tajima K, Hamajima N et al. A large-scale, hospital-based case control study of risk factors of breast cancer according to menopausal status. Jpn J Cancer Res 1995; 86:146-154.
9. Frisch RE, Wyshak G, Albright NL et al. Lower prevalence of breast cancer and cancers of the reproductive system among former college athletes compared to nonathletes. Br J Cancer 1985; 52:885-891.
10. Taioli E, Barone J, Wynder EL. A case control study on breast cancer and body mass. The American Health Foundation—Division of Epidemiology. Eur J Cancer 1995; 31A:723-728.
11. Bernstein L, Henderson BE, Hanisch R et al. Physical exercise and reduced risk of breast cancer in young women. J Natl Cancer Inst 1994; 86:1403-1408.
12. Mittendorf R, Longnecker MP, Newcomb PA et al. Strenuous physical activity in young adulthood and risk of breast cancer (United States). Cancer Causes Control 1995; 6:347-353.
13. Paffenbarger RSJ, Lee IM, Wing AL. The influence of physical activity on the incidence of site-specific cancers in college alumni. Adv Exp Med Biol 1992; 322:7-15.

14. Dorgan JF, Brown C, Barrett M et al. Physical activity and risk of breast cancer in the Framingham Heart Study. Am J Epidemiol 1994; 139:662-669.
15. Hoffman-Goetz L, Husted J. Exercise and breast cancer: review and critical analysis of the literature. Can J Appl Physiol 1994; 19:237-252.
16. Friedenreich CM, Rohan TE. A review of physical activity and breast cancer. Epidemiology 1995; 6:311-317.
17. Hoffman-Goetz L, Husted J. Exercise and cancer: do the biology and epidemiology correspond? Exerc Immunol Rev 1995; 1:81-96.
18. Levi F, La-Vecchia C, Negri E et al. Selected physical activities and the risk of endometrial cancer. Br J Cancer 1993; 67:846-851.
19. Sturgeon SR, Brinton LA, Berman ML et al. Past and present physical activity and endometrial cancer risk. Br J Cancer 1993; 68:584-589.
20. Shu XO, Hatch MC, Zheng W et al. Physical activity and risk of endometrial cancer. Epidemiology 1993; 4:342-349.
21. Hanna N, Schneider M. Enhancement of tumor metastasis and suppression of natural killer cell activity by beta-estradiol treatment. J Immunol 1983; 130:974-980.
22. Hoffman-Goetz L, May KM, Arumugam Y. Exercise training and mouse mammary tumor metastasis. Anticancer Res 1994; 14:2627-2632.
23. MacNeil B, Hoffman-Goetz L. Chronic exercise enhances in vivo and in vitro cytotoxic mechanisms of natural immunity in mice. J Appl Physiol 1993; 74(1):388-395.
24. MacNeil B, Hoffman-Goetz L. Exercise training and tumor metastasis in mice: influence of time of exercise onset. Anticancer Res 1993; 13(6A):2085-2088.
25. Woods JA, Davis JM, Mayer EP et al. Effects of exercise on macrophage activation for antitumor cytotoxicity. J Appl Physiol 1994; 76(5):2177-2185.
26. Woods JA, Davis JM, Mayer EP et al. Exercise increases inflammatory macrophage antitumor cytotoxicity. J Appl Physiol 1993; 75(2):879-886.
27. Woods JA, Davis JM, Kohut ML et al. Effects of exercise on the immune response to cancer. Med Sci Sports Exerc 1994; 26(9):1109-1115.
28. Zaridze DG, Boyle P. Cancer of the prostate: epidemiology and aetiology. Br J Urol 1987; 59(6):493-502.
29. Ahluwalia B, Jackson MA, Jones GW et al. Blood hormone profiles in prostate cancer patients in high-risk and low-risk populations. Cancer 1981; 48(10):2267-2273.

30. Adlercreutz H, Harkonen M, Kuoppasalmi K et al. Effect of training on plasma anabolic and catabolic steroid hormones and their response during physical exercise. Int J Sports Med 1986; 7(Suppl 1):27-28.
31. Hackney AC, Sinning WE, Bruot BC. Reproductive hormonal profiles of endurance-trained and untrained males. Med Sci Sports Exerc 1988; 20(1):60-65.
32. Remes K, Kuoppasalmi K, Adlercreutz H. Effect of physical exercise and sleep deprivation on plasma androgen levels: modifying effect of physical fitness. Int J Sports Med 1985; 6(3):131-135.
33. Vena JE, Graham S, Zielezny M et al. Occupational exercise and risk of cancer. Am J Clin Nutr 1987; 45:318-327.
34. Le-Marchand L, Kolonel LN, Yoshizawa CN. Lifetime occupational physical activity and prostate cancer risk. Am J Epidemiol 1991; 133:103-111.
35. Hsing AW, McLaughlin JK, Zheng W et al. Occupation, physical activity, and risk of prostate cancer in Shanghai, People's Republic of China. Cancer Causes Control 1994; 5:136-140.
36. Whittemore AS, Kolonel LN, Wu AH et al. Prostate cancer in relation to diet, physical activity, and body size in blacks, whites, and Asians in the United States and Canada. J Natl Cancer Inst 1995; 87:652-661.
37. Lee IM, Paffenbarger RSJ, Hsieh CC. Physical activity and risk of prostatic cancer among college alumni. Am J Epidemiol 1992; 135:169-179.
38. Yu H, Harris RE, Wynder EL. Case control study of prostate cancer and socioeconomic factors. Prostate 1988; 13:317-325.
39. Andersson SO, Baron J, Wolk A et al. Early life risk factors for prostate cancer: a population-based case control study in Sweden. Cancer Epidemiol Biomarkers Prev 1995; 4:187-192.
40. Sharpe RM, Skakkebæk NE. Are estrogens involved in falling spermcounts and disorders of the male reproductive tract? Lancet 1993; 341:1392-1395.
41. United Kingdom Testicular Cancer Study Group. Anonymous Aetiology of testicular cancer: association with congenital abnormalities, age at puberty, infertility, and exercise. Br Med J 1994; 308:1393-1399.
42. Gallagher RP, Huchcroft S, Phillips N et al. Physical activity, medical history, and risk of testicular cancer (Alberta and British Columbia, Canada). Cancer Causes Control 1995; 6:398-406.
43. Thune I, Lund E. Physical activity and the risk of prostate and testicular cancer: a cohort study of 53,000 Norwegian men. Cancer Causes Control 1994; 5:549-556.

44. Walker AR, Walker BF, Segal I. Can the risk of colon cancer be lessened? Dig Dis 1993; 11(6):325-333.
45. Persky V, Dyer AR, Leonas J et al. Heart Rate: A Risk Factor for Cancer? Am J Epidemiol 1981; 114:477-487.
46. Garabrant DH, Peters JM, Mack TM et al. Job activity and colon cancer risk. Am J Epidemiol 1984; 119(6):1005-1014.
47. Vena JE, Graham S, Zielezny M et al. Lifetime occupational exercise and colon cancer. Am J Epidemiol 1985; 122:357-365.
48. Fraser G, Pearce N. Occupational physical activity and risk of cancer of the colon and rectum in New Zealand males. Cancer Causes Control 1993; 4:45-50.
49. Chow WH, Dosemeci M, Zheng W et al. Physical activity and occupational risk of colon cancer in Shanghai, China. Int J Epidemiol 1993; 22:23-29.
50. Whittemore AS, Wu-Williams AH, Lee M et al. Diet, physical activity, and colorectal cancer among Chinese in North America and China. J Natl Cancer Inst 1990; 82:915-926.
51. Gerhardsson M, Norell SE, Kiviranta H et al. Sedentary jobs and colon cancer. Am J Epidemiol.1986; 123:775-780.
52. Lynge E, Mellemgaard A, Valentin D et al. Stillesiddende arbejde og kræft. Maanedsskr Prakt Laegegern 1989; tema:861-865.
53. Gerhardsson M, Floderus B, Norell SE. Physical activity and colon cancer risk. Int J Epidemiol 1988; 17:743-746.
54. Markowitz S, Morabia A, Garibaldi K et al. Effect of occupational and recreational activity on the risk of colorectal cancer among males: a case control study. Int J Epidemiol 1992; 21:1057-1062.
55. Kune GA, Kune S, Watson LF. Body weight and physical activity as predictors of colorectal cancer risk. Nutr Cancer 1990; 13:9-17.
56. Slattery ML, Abd-Elghany N, Kerber R et al. Physical activity and colon cancer: a comparison of various indicators of physical activity to evaluate the association. Epidemiology 1990; 1:481-485.
57. Slattery ML, Schumacher MC, Smith KR et al. Physical activity, diet, and risk of colon cancer in Utah. Am J Epidemiol 1988; 128:989-999.
58. Peters RK, Garabrant DH, Yu MC et al. A case control study of occupational and dietary factors in colorectal cancer in young men by subsite. Cancer Res 1989; 49:5459-5468.
59. Arbman G, Axelson O, Fredriksson M et al. Do occupational factors influence the risk of colon and rectal cancer in different ways? Cancer 1993; 72:2543-2549.
60. Fredriksson M, Bengtsson NO, Hardell L et al. Colon cancer, physical activity, and occupational exposures. A case control study. Cancer 1989; 63:1838-1842.

61. Longnecker MP, Gerhardsson-le-Verdier M, Frumkin H et al. A case control study of physical activity in relation to risk of cancer of the right colon and rectum in men. Int J Epidemiol 1995; 24:42-50.
62. Vetter R, Dosemeci M, Blair A et al. Occupational physical activity and colon cancer risk in Turkey. Eur J Epidemiol 1992; 8:845-850.
63. Gerhardsson-de-Verdier M, Steineck G, Hagman U et al. Physical activity and colon cancer: a case-referent study in Stockholm. Int J Cancer 1990; 46:985-989.
64. Jarebinski M, Vlajinac H, Adanja B. Biosocial and other characteristics of the large bowel cancer patients in Belgrade (Yugoslavia). Arch Geschwulstforsch 1988; 58:411-417.
65. Thun MJ, Calle EE, Namboodiri MM et al. Risk factors for fatal colon cancer in a large prospective study [see comments]. J Natl Cancer Inst 1992; 84:1491-1500.
66. Kotake K, Koyama Y, Nasu J et al. Relation of family history of cancer and environmental factors to the risk of colorectal cancer: a case control study. Jpn J Clin Oncol 1995; 25:195-202.
67. Vineis P, Ciccone G, Magnino A. Asbestos exposure, physical activity and colon cancer: a case control study. Tumori 1993; 79:301-303.
68. Brownson RC, Zahm SH, Chang JC et al. Occupational risk of colon cancer. An analysis by anatomic subsite. Am J Epidemiol 1989; 130:675-687.
69. Severson RK, Nomura AM, Grove JS et al. A prospective analysis of physical activity and cancer. Am J Epidemiol 1989; 130:522-529.
70. Giovannucci E, Ascherio A, Rimm EB et al. Physical activity, obesity, and risk for colon cancer and adenoma in men. Ann Intern Med 1995; 122:327-334.
71. Wu AH, Paganini-Hill A, Ross RK et al. Alcohol, physical activity and other risk factors for colorectal cancer: a prospective study. Br J Cancer 1987; 55:687-694.
72. Lee IM, Paffenbarger RSJ, Hsieh C. Physical activity and risk of developing colorectal cancer among college alumni. J Natl Cancer Inst 1991; 83:1324-1329.
73. Lee IM, Paffenbarger RSJ. Physical activity and its relation to cancer risk: a prospective study of college alumni. Med Sci Sports Exerc 1994; 26:831-837.
74. Ballard-Barbash R, Schatzkin A, Albanes D et al. Physical activity and risk of large bowel cancer in the Framingham Study. Cancer Res 1990; 50:3610-3613.
75. Marcus PM, Newcomb PA, Storer BE. Early adulthood physical activity and colon cancer risk among Wisconsin women. Cancer Epidemiol Biomarkers Prev 1994; 3:641-644.

76. Hoffman-Goetz L. 10, Exercise, Immunity, and colon cancer. In: Hoffman-Goetz L, Husted J, eds. Exercise and Immune Function. New York: CRC Press, 1996:179-198.
77. Macfarlane GJ, Lowenfels AB. Physical activity and colon cancer. Eur J Cancer Prev 1994; 3:393-398.
78. Sutherland WH, Nye ER, Macfarlane DJ et al. Fecal bile acid concentration in distance runners. Int J Sports Med 1991; 12:533-536.
79. Ravikumar T, Rodrick M, Steele GJ et al. Interleukin generation in experimental colon cancer of rats: effects of tumor growth and tumor therapy. J Natl Cancer Inst 1985; 74:893-898.
80. Hoffman M, Pollack S. In: Oppenheim JJ, Cohen S, eds. Inteleukins, Lymphokines and Cytokines. New York: Academic Press, 1983:707p.
81. Fielding RA, Manfredi TJ, Ding W et al. Acute phase response in exercise. III. Neutrophil and IL-1 beta accumulation in skeletal muscle. Am J Physiol 1993; 265(1 Pt 2):R166-172.
82. Cannon JG, Fielding RA, Fiatarone MA et al. Increased interleukin 1 beta in human skeletal muscle after exercise. Am J Physiol 1989; 257(2 Pt 2):R451-455.
83. Northoff H, Berg A. Immunologic mediators as parameters of the reaction to strenuous exercise. Int J Sports Med 1991; 12(Suppl 1):S9-15.
84. Rivier A, Pene J, Chanez P et al. Release of cytokines by blood monocytes during strenuous exercise. Int J Sports Med 1994; 15(4):192-198.
85. Cannon JG, Evans WJ, Hughes VA et al. Physiological mechanisms contributing to increased interleukin-1 secretion. J Appl Physiol 1986; 61(5):1869-1874.
86. Espersen GT, Elbaek A, Ernst E et al. Effect of physical exercise on cytokines and lymphocyte subpopulations in human peripheral blood. APMIS 1990; 98(5):395-400.
87. Evans WJ, Meredith CN, Cannon JG et al. Metabolic changes following eccentric exercise in trained and untrained men. J Appl Physiol 1986; 61:1864-1868.
88. Cannon JG. Exercise and the acute phase response. In: Hoffman-Goetz L, ed. Exercise and Immune Function. New York: CRC Press, 1996:39-54.
89. Haahr PM, Pedersen BK, Fomsgaard A et al. Effect of physical exercise on in vitro production of interleukin 1, interleukin 6, tumor necrosis factor-alpha, interleukin 2 and interferon-gamma. Int J Sports Med 1991; 12(2):223-7.
90. Clemmensen IH, Storm HH. Cancer in Denmark 1993. Copenhagen: Danish Cancer Society, 1996.

91. Lindblad P, Wolk A, Bergstrom R et al. The role of obesity and weight fluctuations in the etiology of renal cell cancer: a population-based case control study. Cancer Epidemiol Biomarkers Prev 1994; 3:631-639.
92. Mellemgaard A, Lindblad P, Schlehofer B et al. International renal-cell cancer study. III. Role of weight, height, physical activity, and use of amphetamines. Int J Cancer 1995; 60:350-354.
93. Mellemgaard A, Engholm G, McLaughlin JK et al. Risk factors for renal-cell carcinoma in Denmark. III. Role of weight, physical activity and reproductive factors. Int J Cancer 1994; 56:66-71.
94. Goodman MT, Morgenstern H, Wynder EL. A case control study of factors affecting the development of renal cell cancer. Am J Epidemiol 1986; 124:926-941.
95. Stukonis M, Doll R. Gastric cancer in man and physical activity at work. Int J Cancer 1969; 4:248-254.
96. Nomura AM, Stemmermann GN, Chyou PH. Gastric cancer among the Japanese in Hawaii. Jpn J Cancer Res 1995; 86:916-923.
97. Frentzel-Beyme R, Chang-Claude J. Vegetarian diets and colon cancer: the German experience. Am J Clin Nutr 1994; 59:1143S-1152S.
98. Wannamethee G, Shaper AG, Macfarlane PW. Heart rate, physical activity, and mortality from cancer and other noncardiovascular diseases. Am J Epidemiol 1993; 137:735-748.
99. Brownson RC, Chang JC, Davis JR et al. Physical activity on the job and cancer in Missouri. Am J Public Health 1991; 81:639-642.
100. Garfinkel L, Stellman SD. Mortality by relative weight and exercise. Cancer 1988; 62:1844-1850.
101. Garfinkel L, Heath CWJ. Cancer prevention study II: The American Cancer Society prospective study. Statistical Bulletin 1992; 21-29.
102. Albanes D, Blair A, Taylor PR. Physical activity and risk of cancer in the NHANES I population. Am J Public Health 1989; 79:744-750.
103. Polednak AP. College athletics, body size, and cancer mortality. Cancer 1976; 38:382-387.
104. Blair SN, Kohl HW, Paffenbarger RSJ et al. Physical fitness and all-cause mortality. A prospective study of healthy men and women. JAMA 1989; 262:2395-2401.
105. Pukkala E, Poskiparta M, Apter D et al. Life-long physical activity and cancer risk among Finnish female teachers. Eur J Cancer Prev 1993; 2:369-376.
106. Frisch RE, Wyshak G, Albright NL et al. Lower prevalence of nonreproductive system cancers among female former college athletes. Med Sci Sports Exerc 1989; 21:250-253.

107. Hoffman-Goetz L, Pedersen BK. Exercise and the immune system: a model of the stress response? Immunol Today 1994; 15(8):382-387.
108. Thomas L. Discussion; reactions to homologous tissue antigens. In: Lawrence HS, ed. Cellular and Humoral Aspects of the Hypersensitive States. London: Cassel, 1959:529-532.
109. Burnet FM. Somatic mutation and chronic disease. Br Med J 1965; 1:338-342.
110. Burnet FM. Immunological factors in the process of carcinogenesis. Br Med Bull 1964; 20:154-158.
111. Kinlein LJ. Immunosuppression and cancer. In: Vainio H, Magee PN, McGregor DB et al, eds. Mechanisms of Carcinogenesis in Risk Identification. Lyon: IARC, 1992:237-253.
112. Levine AM. AIDS-related malignancies:the emerging epidemic. J Natl Cancer Inst 1993; 85:1382-1397.
113. Birkeland SA, Storm H, Lamm LU et al. Cancer after renal transplantation in the nordic countries, 1964-1986. Int J Cancer 1995; 60:183-189.
114. Chang Y, Cesarman E, Pessin MS et al. Identification of herpesvirus-like DNA sequences in AIDS-associated Kaposi's sarcoma. Science 1994; 266(5192):1865-1869.
115. The EUROGAST Study Group. An international association between helicobacter pylori infection and gastric cancer. Lancet 1993; 341:1359-1362.
116. Pedersen BK, Ullum H. NK cell response to physical activity: possible mechanisms of action. Med Sci Sports Exerc 1994; 26(2):140-146.
117. Brines R, Hoffman-Goetz L, Pedersen BK. Can you exercise to make your immune system fitter? Immunol Today 1996; 17(6):252-254.
118. Fitzgerald L. Exercise and the immune system. Immunol Today 1988; 9(11):337-339.
119. Clemmensen IH, Storm HH. Exessive physical activity and cancer risk, abstract. Int J Sports Med 1996; (in press).

INDEX